It's Hard To Believe With No Salt No Sugar

by

E L Hughes

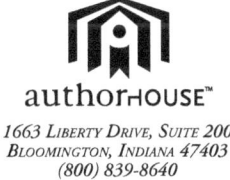

1663 LIBERTY DRIVE, SUITE 200
BLOOMINGTON, INDIANA 47403
(800) 839-8640
WWW.AUTHORHOUSE.COM

First published by AuthorHouse 07/27/05

ISBN: 1-4208-6279-0 (sc)

Library of Congress Control Number: 2005903032

Printed in the United States of America
Bloomington, Indiana

This book is printed on acid-free paper.

THIS BOOK IS YOUR NEW COOKING GUIDE

The sole purpose of this book is to assist you in preparing your families favorite meals without adding salt or sugar yet bursting with deep flavor.

With the use of our special seasoning and baking methods, your family will be able to enjoy the same meals you have grown accustomed, with the exception of the dangerous effects of salt and sugar.

Meal time will now become more satisfying and healthier for the entire family.

REMEMBER: Most packaged foods contain some sodium (salt) and sugar, so read your labels very carefully. Try to find the products with the least amount of salt or sugar.

Contents

Health Charts

THE NUMBER OF SERVINGS
PER DAY

===

Lean Meats-------------------------4 to 6 oz.---------------------Servings per day

Raw Vegetables------------------3 to 5----------------------------Servings per day

Cooked Vegetables-------------3 to 5----------------------------Servings per day

Starchy Vegetables------------6 to 8----------------------------Servings per day

Fruit------------------------------------2 to 4----------------------------Servings per day

Sweets-------------------------------1 to 2----------------------------Servings per day

===

These are recommended servings per day,
check with your doctor or registered dietitian
for *your* individual number of servings per day. (6)

Rate Your Plate Chart

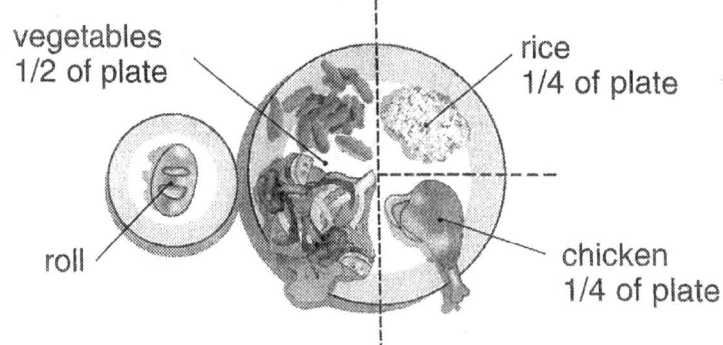

vegetables
1/2 of plate

rice
1/4 of plate

roll

chicken
1/4 of plate

DAILY INTAKE

Percent daily values are based on a 2,000 and 2,500 calorie intake per day. Your daily values may be higher or lower depending on your calorie needs.

Calories:	2,000/day	2,500/day
Total Fat	50g	62g
Saturated Fat	12g	15g
Cholesterol	200g	200g
Sodium	2000g	2400g
Carbohydrate	150g	180g

This is a recommended daily intake. Make sure you check with your doctor for your daily intake. (5)

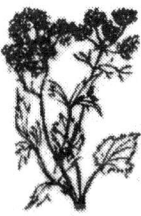

CHOLESTEROL CHART

	Desirable	Borderline (high)	High Risk
Total Cholesterol	<200	200-240	>240
Low Density Cholesterol	<130	130-160	>240
High Density Cholesterol	>50	50-35	<35
Triglycerides	<150	150-500	>500

Note:

Cholesterol and Triglycerides together constitutes blood lipids and fats.

High density cholesterols (HDL) are considered good cholesterol and reduces harmful low density cholesterol from the blood and tissue and delivers it to the liver where it is processed for excretion.

Low density cholesterols (LDL) promote deposits in the arteries gradually leading to narrowing and hardening which blocks the passage of blood. This condition is termed as "artherosclerosis" which leads to high blood pressure and heart diseases.

Sedentary life style decreases energy spending by the body and contributes to over weight and rise in blood lipids. Exercise increases good cholesterol (HDL). [2]

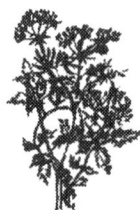

BLOOD PRESSURE CHART

Category	Systolic BP (mmHg)	Diastolic BP (mmHg)	Follow-up Recommendations
Optimal	less than 120	less than 80	Recheck in 2 years
Normal	less than 130	less than 85	Recheck in 2 years
High-normal	130-139	85-89	Recheck in 1 year
Hypertension			
Stage 1	140-159	90-99	Confirm within 2 months
Stage 2	160-179	100-109	Evaluate within 1 month
Stage 3	180 and above	110 and above	Evaluate immediately or within 1 week, depending on the clinical situation

BLOOD PRESSURE

"Blood pressure" is actually the force that is exerted against the artery walls as blood is carried through the circulatory system. It is recorded as a measurement of this force in relation to the heart's pumping activity, and is measured in millimeters of mercury (mmHg). The top number or systolic pressure is the measurement of the pressure that occurs when the heart contracts or beats. The bottom number or diastolic pressure is the measurement recorded between beats, while the heart is at rest. The systolic number is placed over the diastolic number. An example would be 110/70 (read as 110 over 70). The systolic number is always the higher of the two numbers.

ELEVATED LEVELS

Hypertension is an indicator that the force required for blood flow is greater than normal. According to the new Sixth Report of the Joint National Committee on Detection, Evaluation, and Treatment of High Blood Pressure (JNC VI), a blood pressure measurement of less than 130/85 is considered "normal"; 130-140/85-90 is defined as "high normal".

Blood pressure is considered to be elevated when repeated measurement is greater than 140/90 of either the systolic, diastolic, or both measurements. A diagnosis of hypertension is made when a person has had 2 or more elevated readings after the initial assessment.

JNC VI BLOOD PRESSURE CHART

The Sixth Report of the Joint National Committee on Prevention, Detection, Evaluation and Treatment of High Blood Pressure has published the following chart to classify blood pressure. The chart applies to patients who are 18 years and older, who have not already been diagnosed with hypertension, are not on any medication for hypertension, and are not seriously ill [1]

DIABETES CHART

It is recommended that you have a HbA1c test, which is usually given quarterly in your doctor's office. It shows your average blood glucose level over the previous three months and can be used to predict your risk for diabetes complications.

Use the chart below to compare your daily blood glucose test results to your quarterly HbA1c results. With this information, you and your doctor can determine how well your diabetes is being controlled. (3)

COMPARING BLOOD GLUCOSE WITH HBA1C

Average Glucose, mg/dL		HbA1c, %
90 120	Excellent	5 6
150 180	Good	7 8
210 240	Fair	9 10
270 300	Poor	11 12

Average Glucose, mg/dL   HbA1c, %

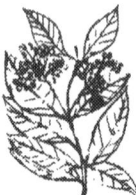

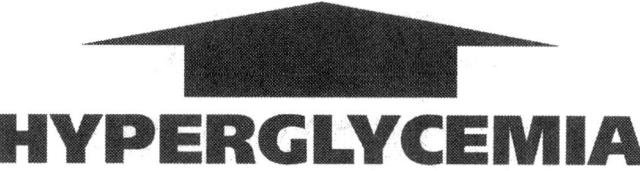

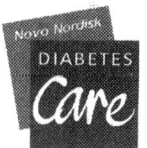

HYPERGLYCEMIA
(High Blood Glucose)

Causes: Too much food, too little insulin or diabetes medicine, illness or stress.

Onset: Gradual, may progress to diabetic coma.

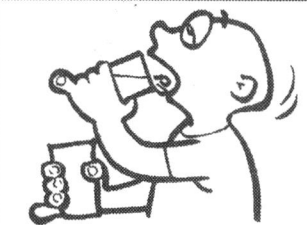

EXTREME THIRST

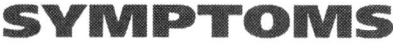

SYMPTOMS

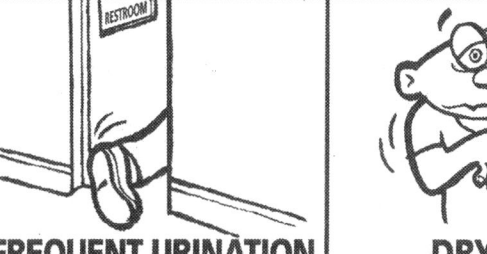

FREQUENT URINATION

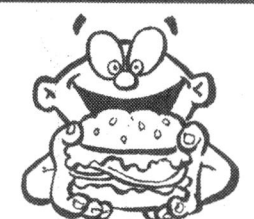

DRY SKIN

HUNGER

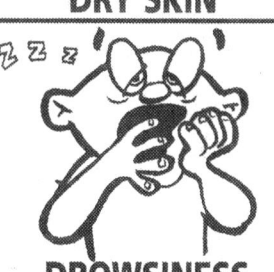

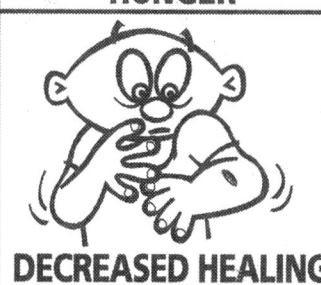

BLURRED VISION

DROWSINESS

DECREASED HEALING

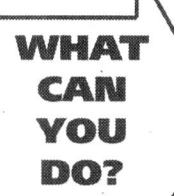

WHAT CAN YOU DO?

TEST BLOOD GLUCOSE

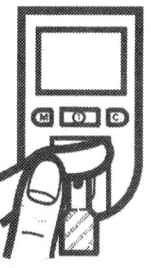

If over 200 mg/dL for several tests or for 2 days

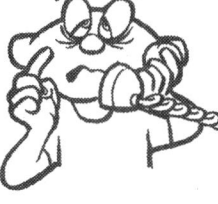

CALL YOUR DOCTOR

Concept developed by Rhoda Rogers, RN, BSN, CDE, Sunrise Community Health Center, Greeley, Colorado
©1999 Novo Nordisk Pharmaceuticals, Inc.   000-114   Printed in U.S.A.

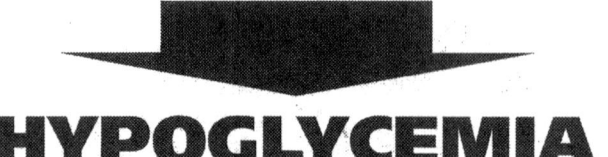

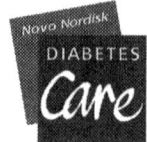
HYPOGLYCEMIA
(Low Blood Glucose)

Causes: Too little food, too much insulin or diabetes medicine, or extra activity.

Onset: Sudden, may progress to insulin shock.

SYMPTOMS

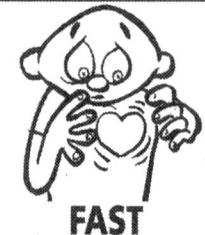

SHAKING

FAST HEARTBEAT

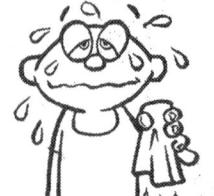

SWEATING

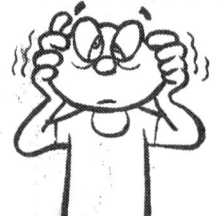

DIZZINESS

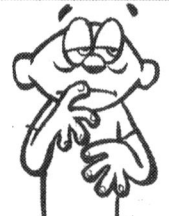

ANXIOUS

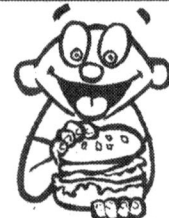

HUNGER

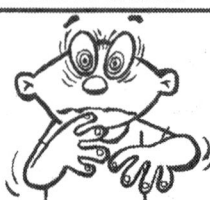

IMPAIRED VISION

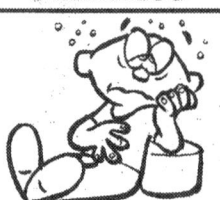

WEAKNESS FATIGUE

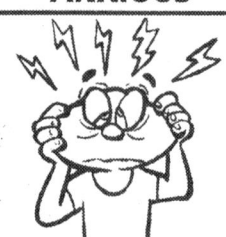

HEADACHE

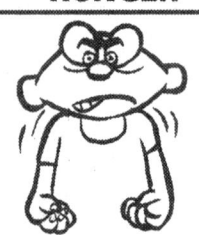

IRRITABLE

WHAT CAN YOU DO?

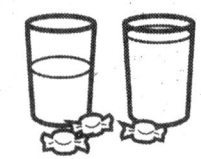

Drink 1/2 glass of juice or regular soft drink, or 1 glass of milk, or eat some soft candies (not chocolate).

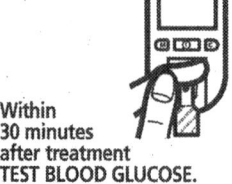

Within 30 minutes after treatment TEST BLOOD GLUCOSE. If symptoms don't stop, call your doctor

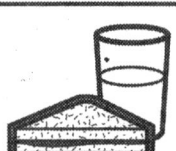

Then, eat a light snack (1/2 peanut butter or meat sandwich and 1/2 glass of milk).

Treatment may vary with different medications.

Concept developed by Rhoda Rogers, RN, BSN, CDE, Sunrise Community Health Center, Greeley, Colorado
©1999 Novo Nordisk Pharmaceuticals, Inc.   000-114   Printed in U.S.A.

Proper Foot Care

Proper foot care is an important part of diabetes management.
To avoid serious problems, follow these important self-care tips:

Check Your Feet Daily

Check the tops and bottoms of your feet, especially between your toes.
If you can't see the bottoms, use a mirror.

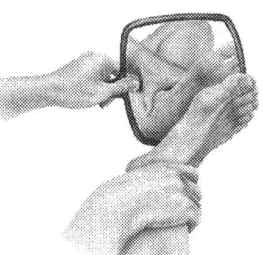

LOOK FOR:

- Skin color changes
- Pain in legs
- Ingrown or fungal toenails
- Corns or calluses
- Swelling of foot or ankle
- Open sores that are slow to heal
- Dry cracks in the skin

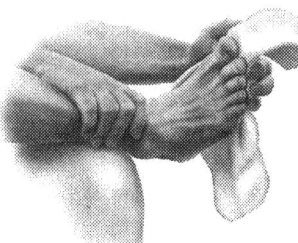

Wash Your Feet Daily

- Wash your feet with mild soap and lukewarm water in the morning or before you go to bed.

- Gently dry your feet with a soft towel, especially between the toes.

- Use moisturizing lotion (not between toes) to keep skin from cracking.

Cut Toenails Regularly

- Cut your toenails straight across. Use toenail clippers with a straight edge.

- Never cut into corners. This could trigger an ingrown toenail.

- Cut your toenails after bathing, when they are easiest to trim.

See your healthcare provider immediately if you recognize any foot problems.

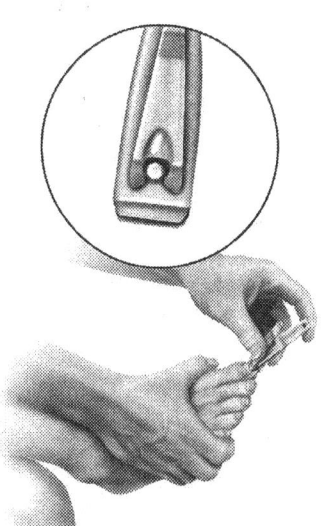

Proper Footwear

Proper footwear plays a major role in preventing foot problems associated with diabetes.
Follow these tips before buying or putting on a pair of shoes:

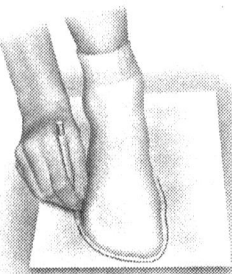

Measure Your Feet

The size and shape of your feet can change over time. Have your
feet measured before buying a new pair. If an experienced shoe
fitter is not around, you can fit yourself. Here's how:

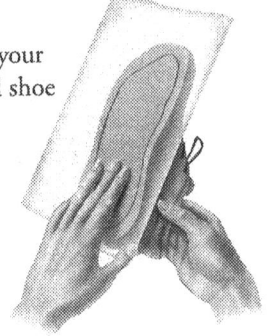

1. Trace an outline of your foot on a piece of paper.
2. Place the shoe over the outline.

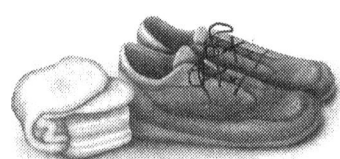

Choose the Right Shoes

- New shoes should be sturdy and comfortable. They must fit the length
  and width of the foot (leave room for toes to wiggle).

- Always wear socks or stockings with your shoes. Socks made of wool or
  100% cotton offer the most protection. They also keep your feet
  warm and dry.

- Break in new shoes slowly by wearing them for only one or
  two hours at a time.

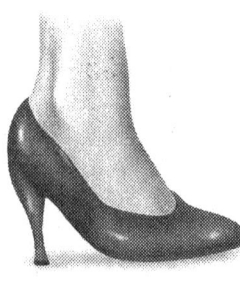

Things to Avoid:

- Do not wear high heels, sandals, and pointed-toe shoes. They put excess
  pressure on your feet.

- Do not walk barefoot, even in your home or at the beach.

- Do not wear mended or seamed socks. They can cause blisters or
  skin injuries.

- Do not wear nylon stockings if you're being treated for an infection.

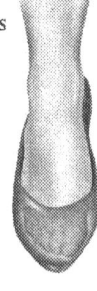

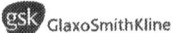

Weight Chart For Female

Height	Age 17-20	Age 21-27	Age 28-39	Age 40+
4'8"	109	112	115	119
4'9"	113	116	119	123
4'10"	116	120	123	127
4'11"	120	124	127	131
5'0"	125	129	132	137
5'1"	129	133	137	141
5'2"	133	137	141	145
5'3"	137	141	145	149
5'4"	141	148	150	154
5'5"	145	149	154	159
5'6"	150	154	159	164
5'7"	154	158	163	168
5'8"	159	163	168	173
5'9"	163	167	172	177
5'10"	167	172	177	183
5'11"	172	177	182	188
6'0"	178	183	189	194
6'1"	183	188	194	200
6'2"	189	194	200	206
6'3"	193	199	205	211
6'4"	198	204	210	216
6'5"	203	209	215	222
6'6"	208	214	220	227

Note:

a. If the height fraction is less than 1/2 inch, round down to the nearest whole number in inches.

b. If the height fraction is 1/2 inch or greater, round up to the next highest whole number in inches. (4)

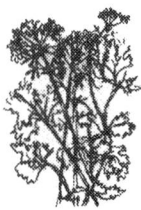

11

Weight Chart For Males

Height	Age 17-20	Age 21-27	Age 28-39	Age 40+
4'10"	132	136	139	141
4'11"	136	140	144	146
5'0"	141	144	148	150
5'1"	145	149	153	155
5'2"	150	154	158	160
5'3"	155	159	163	165
5'4"	160	163	168	170
5'5"	165	169	174	178
5'6"	170	174	179	181
5'7"	175	179	184	186
5'8"	180	185	189	192
5'9"	185	189	194	197
5'10"	190	195	200	203
5'11"	195	200	205	208
6'0"	201	206	211	214
6'1"	206	212	217	220
6'2"	212	217	223	226
6'3"	218	223	229	232
6'4"	223	229	235	238
6'5"	229	235	241	244
6'6"	234	240	247	250

Note:

a. If the height fraction is less than 1/2 inch, round down to the nearest whole number in inches.

b. If the height fraction is 1/2 inch or greater, round up to the next highest whole number in inches. (4)

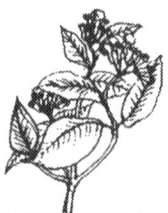

HOUSE SEASONING
(Salt Replacement)

4 Tbsp	-	Onion Powder
4 Tbsp	-	Garlic Powder
4 Tbsp	-	Chili Powder
4 Tbsp	-	Paprika
2 Tbsp	-	Basil
2 Tbsp	-	Lemon Peel
2 Tbsp	-	Minced Garlic (dry)
2 Tbsp	-	Oregano
2 Tbsp	-	Splenda Sugar Blend for Baking
1 Tbsp	-	Cayenne Pepper
4 Cubes	-	Chicken Bouillon (Crushed)

Preparation:

1. Place bouillon cubes in a paper towel; with a large spoon or the back of a knife lightly crush until cubes become powdery.

2. In a large measuring cup or bowl combine all the above ingredients including bouillon cube powder. Mix with spoon until well blended.

3. Pour in a large shaker with large holes.

4. Replace the salt in your kitchen with this recipe.

5. Makes approx 2 cups.

IMPORTANT: All ingredients can be founded in your local Dollar Store or Grocery Store.

Or Order At: www.nosaltnosugar.com

HOUSE RULES

1.	**Vegetables**	-	Never use can vegetables. Always use frozen or fresh.
2.	**Salt & Sugar**	-	You are allowed a maximum of 2400 mg of sodium which means SALT per day. Do not add salt or sugar to your prepared food.
3.	**Dessert**	-	Keep a healthy sweet snack on hand. This will eliminate eating the wrong foods.
4.	**Fresh Fruit**	-	Fresh fruit is great for snacking and you are allowed 2 to 4 servings per day.
5.	**Preparing Food**	-	Use low sodium chicken broth, light margarine, splenda sugar and house seasoning.
6.	**Seasoning Food**	-	It is important to keep house seasoning on hand at all times.
7.	**Candy**	-	Buy sugar free candy or make your own.
8.	**Pasta, Rice & Potatoes**	-	Boil with light margarine and chicken bouillon cubes.

This is not a diet book but, a cookbook designed to allow your entire family to enjoy everyday foods with an incredible taste. Our cookbook allows the family members who are diagnosed with high blood pressure, heart disease, diabetes and cholesterol to enjoy the same foods the rest of the family enjoys

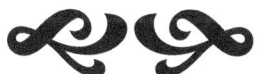

Salads & Fruits

CHICKEN & LETTUCE SALAD

2	-	Chicken Breast Halves
1 Bag	-	Lettuce (your choice)
10	-	Cherry Tomatoes
3 Tbsp.	-	Parmesan Cheese (in jar)
1 Tbsp.	-	Low Fat Oil
2 Tbsp.	-	House Seasoning

Preparation:

1. Remove skin and any excess fat from breast, slice in strips wash and add house seasoning.

2. Heat large skillet with oil. Add breast strips, cook until strips are completely tender, turning occasionally. Remove from heat.

3. Cut tomatoes in halves. On large plate, layer lettuce, tomatoes and chicken strips. Sprinkle parmesan cheese over salad and serve.

Recommend 1 Cup per serving

===

LETTUCE SALAD

1/2	-	Head Lettuce
2	-	Eggs
1 Lg.	-	Tomato
1	-	Avocado
1	-	Red Bell Pepper
1/2 Cup	-	Cheddar Cheese (Reduced Fat)

Preparation:

1. Boil eggs, cut up tomatoes, avocado and eggs. In large bowl, layer lettuce, avocado, tomatoes, bell pepper, eggs and sprinkle top with shredded cheese.

2. Serve with low fat or light dressing.

Recommend 1 Cup per serving

CHICKEN OR TURKEY SALAD

2	-	Chicken Breast or any parts
3 Cups	-	Water
2 Tbsp.	-	Light Margarine
3 Tbsp.	-	Light Mayonnaise
2 Tbsp.	-	Pickle Relish
1/4	-	Onion (chopped)
3	-	Eggs (boiled)
2	-	Chicken Bouillon Cubes
1 Tbsp	-	House Seasoning

Preparation:

1. Remove skin and add house seasoning, margarine, bouillon cubes and water in large pot. Boil until tender, remove and cut in small pieces. Boil eggs.

2. Cut up eggs and onion in small pieces. In large bowl combine chicken and remaining ingredients. Mix well.

Recommend 1/2 Cup per serving

==

TURKEY TACO SALAD

1 Lb.	-	Ground Turkey
1 Tbsp.	-	House Seasoning
1 Can	-	Stewed Tomatoes (Low Sodium)
1/2 Head	-	Lettuce (Shredded)
1 Cup	-	Cheddar Cheese (Reduced Fat)
1/2	-	Onion (Thinly Sliced)

Preparation:

1. In large skillet, add turkey, house seasoning and 1/4 onion. Cook until turkey is tender. Add tomatoes and simmer for additional 5 min. Remove from heat and set aside.

2. On large plate, layer lettuce, 1/2 cheese and remaining onion. With large spoon carefully spoon turkey mixture over lettuce. Sprinkle remaining cheese over top of salad.

Recommend 1/2 Cup per serving

EGG SALAD

4	-	Eggs (Boiled)
2 Tbsp.	-	Light Mayonnaise
1 Tbsp.	-	Pickle Relish

Preparation:

1. Boil eggs, peel and dice into small pieces. In medium bowl combine all the above ingredients. Mix well.

2. Serve on wheat crackers or wheat bread.

Recommend 1/3 Cup per serving

==

SHRIMP & PEA SALAD

1 Lb.	-	Cooked Shrimp
1 Cup	-	Small green peas (Cooked)
1/2	-	Onion (Finely Chopped)
1 Cup	-	Cheddar Cheese (Reduced Fat)
3 Tbsp.	-	Light Mayonnaise

Preparation:

1. Combine shrimp, peas, onion and cheese in medium bowl.

2. Add mayonnaise and gently toss until mayonnaise covers entire mixture. Chill and Serve.

Recommend 1/2 Cup per serving

BAG COLESLAW

1 (8 oz Bag)	-	Coleslaw
1/4	-	Onion (Sliced)
1/2 Tsp.	-	Splenda Sugar Blend for Baking
3 Tbsp.	-	Light Mayonnaise

Preparation:

1. In medium bowl combine coleslaw, thinly sliced onion, splenda and mayonnaise. Toss making sure slaw is coated with mayonnaise.

2. Serve at room temperature or chilled.

Recommend 1/2 Cup per serving

===

COLESLAW

1	-	Head Cabbage (Shredded)
1/2	-	Red Bell Pepper
1/2	-	Green Bell Pepper
1/2	-	Onion (Thinly Sliced)
2 Tsp.	-	Splenda Sugar Blend for Baking
1/2 Cup	-	Light Mayonnaise

Preparation:

1. Shred cabbage and cut up peppers and onions. In large bowl, mix cabbage, peppers, onion, splenda and mayonnaise. Blend until well coated and serve.

Recommend 1/2 Cup per serving

POTATO SALAD

2 Lg.	-	White Potatoes
3 Cups	-	Water
2 Tbsp.	-	Light Margarine
2	-	Chicken Bouillon Cubes
3 Tbsp.	-	Light Mayonnaise
2 Tbsp.	-	Pickle Relish
3	-	Eggs (Boiled)
1/4	-	Onion
1 Tsp.	-	Splenda Sugar Blend for Baking

Preparation:

1. Peel and dice potatoes, add water, margarine, bouillon cubes and boil until tender. Drain and set aside. Boil eggs.

2. Cut up eggs and onion in small pieces. In large bowl combine potatoes and remaining ingredients. Toss to blend (do not beat). Serve warm or cold.

Recommend 1/3 Cup per serving

==

CABBAGE SALAD

2	-	Large Apples (grated)
1 Cup	-	Carrots (grated)
2 Cups	-	Cabbage (grated)
1/2 Cup	-	Raisins (optional)
1 Cup	-	Celery (chopped in small pieces)
4 Tbsp.	-	Light Mayonnaise

Preparation:

1. Grate apples, carrots and cabbage. Chop celery in large bowl, add remaining ingredients and toss until mayonnaise has coated entire salad. Serve warm or cold.

Recommend 1 Cup per serving

CUCUMBER SALAD

3 med.	-	Cucumbers (Peeled & thinly sliced)
1/2 Cup	-	Green Onions (Chopped)
1 Tbsp.	-	Lemon Juice
1/3 Cup	-	Sour Cream (Fat Free)
2 Tsp.	-	Splenda Sugar Blend for Baking

Preparation:

1. Peel and cut cucumbers in thin slices. Add chopped onions, lemon juice and splenda sugar.

2. Toss and refrigerate. Just before serving add sour cream and toss making sure cucumbers are well coated.

Recommend 1 Cup per serving

==

BANANA SALAD

2	-	Bananas (Sliced)
2	-	Peaches
8	-	Dates (Cut in small pieces)
4	-	Slices Pineapples (Packed in own juice)
2	-	Large Lettuce Leaves
1 Tsp.	-	Splenda Sugar Blend for Baking

Preparation:

1. Place lettuce leaves on plate. Layer pineapples, bananas, peaches and dates.

2. Mix 1/3 Cup of pineapple juice with 1 Tsp. splenda sugar, mix well. Pour over banana layers and serve.

Recommend 1 Cup per serving

FRESH FRUIT SALAD

1 Cup	-	Sliced Strawberries
1 Cup	-	Cubed Cantaloupe
1 Cup	-	Cubed Watermelon
1 Cup	-	Cubed Honeydew Melon
1 Cup	-	Sliced Peaches
1 Cup	-	Seedless Grapes
1 Cup	-	Cubed Apples
1 Tsp.	-	Splenda Sugar Blend for Baking
1 Cup	-	Orange Juice

Preparation:

1. In large bowl, cut up all fruit.

2. Mix orange juice and Splenda. Pour over fruit and mix well. Chill 1 to 2 hours before erving.

Recommend 1 Cup per serving

==

SUMMER BERRIES

4 Cups	-	Raspberries
2 Cups	-	Blueberries
2 Cups	-	Blackberries
2 Tbsp.	-	Splenda Sugar Blend for Baking
1 Tbsp.	-	Lemon Juice

Preparation:

1. Sort and wash all berries. Combine all ingredients in large bowl and gently mix until combined.

2. Let fruit stand at room temperature stirring occasionally for 15 min. Serve chilled or at room temperature.

Recommend 1 Cup per serving

PEACHES & CREAM

6	-	Peaches (Sliced)
1/2 Cup	-	Heavy Cream
1 Tsp.	-	Splenda Sugar Blend for Baking

Preparation:

1. Slice peaches in medium bowl. Mix splenda sugar and heavy cream. Pour mixture over peaches.

2. Toss to coat peaches chill and serve.

Recommend 1 Cup per serving

==

STRAWBERRIES & CREAM

1 Pint	-	Fresh Strawberries
1/2 Cup	-	Heavy Cream
1 Tsp.	-	Splenda Sugar Blend for Baking
1/2 Tsp.	-	Cinnamon (Optional)

Preparation:

1. Wash and cut up strawberries. Place in large bowl. In small bowl, mix cream and splenda.

2. Pour cream mixture over berries and toss to coat with cream. (Optional: Sprinkle with cinnamon.)

Recommend 1 Cup per serving

BANANA SMOOTHIE

2	-	Bananas (Frozen, Peel Before Freezing)
1 Cup	-	Apple Juice (Unsweetened)
4	-	Strawberries (Frozen)
1/2 Tsp.	-	Splenda Sugar Blend for Baking

Preparation:

1. Peel bananas, freeze bananas and strawberries. Pour apple juice and splenda in blender.

2. Cut bananas and strawberries in small pieces and add to blender. Mix to desired consistence and serve.

Recommend 1 (8 oz.) Glass per serving

==

FRESH FRUIT SALAD

3	-	Bananas (Sliced)
2	-	Apples (Sliced)
1	-	Pear (Sliced)
1	-	Peach (Sliced)
8	-	Dates (Cut into small pieces)
1/2 Cup	-	Orange Juice
1/2 Tsp.	-	Splenda Sugar Blend for Baking

Preparation:

1. Slice all fruit in large bowl. Mix orange juice and splenda in a Cup and pour over fruit mixture. Toss making sure all fruit is coated.

2. Chill approx. 1 hour before serving.

Recommend 1 Cup per serving

FRUIT PARFAITS

2 Cups	-	Frozen or Fresh Fruit (Strawberries, Peaches, Raspberries or Blueberries
2 (8 oz.)	-	Carton Lemon Low Fat Yogurt
1 Tsp.	-	Splenda Sugar Blend for Baking

Preparation:

1. In medium bowl add fruit and sprinkle with splenda sugar. Toss to coat fruit. Use 4 parfait glasses or Cups.

2. Layer fruit and yogurt evenly. Begin and end with fruit.

Recommend 1 glass or Cup per serving

==

ORANGE DELIGHT

2 Lg. Cans.	-	Mandarin Orange slices (packed in own juice)
2 Tsp.	-	Splenda Sugar Blend for Baking
1 (8 oz.) Tube	-	Whip Cream (Fat Free Thawed)
1 sm.	-	Apple (Optional)

Preparation:

1. Open and drain orange slices, make sure slices are well drained.

2. In medium bowl sprinkle with splenda sugar. Add thawed whip cream and toss. (Optional: Cut 1 apple and add before tossing.) Chill and serve.

Recommend 1 Cup per serving

Soups and Sauces

GUMBO

2	-	Chicken Breast (or any parts)
5 Cups	-	Water
4	-	Chicken Bouillon Cubes
2 Tbsp.	-	House Seasoning
1 Cup	-	Onion (chopped)
1 Cup	-	Celery (chopped)
1 Tbsp.	-	Hot Sauce
1 Pkg.	-	Frozen Gumbo Blend Vegetables
1 Pkg.	-	Frozen Crawfish (Thawed)
1 Pkg.	-	Frozen Shrimp (Thawed)

Preparation:

1. In large pot add water, chicken, bouillon cubes, onion, celery, house seasoning and hot sauce.

2. Bring to boil, reduce heat and boil until chicken is tender.

3. Remove chicken from pot removing skin and debone. Pull chicken into small pieces and set aside.

4. Add gumbo vegetable mix and boil until tender approx 30 min.

5. Add crawfish, shrimp and chicken, simmer for 5 min. and serve.

Recommend 1 Cup per serving

CHICKEN SOUP

1	-	Chicken (cut-up)
1 Tbsp.	-	House Seasoning
1/2 Cup	-	Onion
1/2 Cup	-	Celery
1/2 Cup	-	Red Bell Pepper
1 Cup	-	Cheddar Cheese (Reduced Fat)
1/2 Cup	-	Heavy Cream
2 Tbsp.	-	Light Margarine
4	-	Chicken Bouillon Cubes
6 Cups	-	Water

Preparation:

1. Boil chicken in water, house seasoning, onion, margarine, celery, bell pepper and bouillon cubes.

2. When done, remove skin and debone, pull chicken apart in large pieces.

3. Add cream, chicken and cheese. Simmer approx. 10 min. or until cheese melts and serve.

Recommend 1 Cup per serving

CRAWFISH WITH SAUCE

1 pkg.	-	Frozen Crawfish (thawed)
1 Cup	-	Chicken Broth (low sodium)
1 Cup	-	Heavy Cream
1 Cup	-	Cheddar Cheese (Reduced Fat)
½ Cup	-	Onion
½ Cup	-	Celery
1 Tbsp.	-	House Seasoning
1 Tbsp.	-	Light Margarine

Preparation:

1. Sauté margarine, onion and celery until tender. Add chicken broth, cream and cheese. Simmer until thick. Add crawfish and house seasoning and simmer approx. 3 min.

2. Serve over rice, pasta or potatoes.

Recommend 1/2 Cup per serving

==

ONION SOUP

2 Lg.	-	Sweet Onion
½ Cup	-	Light Margarine
2 Cans	-	Stewed Tomatoes (Low sodium)
1 Tbsp.	-	House Seasoning
1	-	Chicken Bouillon cube
2 Cups	-	Water

Preparation:

1. Sauté margarine and onion in large saucepan; add tomatoes, water, bouillon cubes and house seasoning. Cover and simmer approx 30 to 40 min.

Recommend 1 Cup per serving

BROCCOLI-CORN CHOWDER SOUP

1 (16 oz.) Pkg.	-	Broccoli (stir fry)
2 Tbsp.	-	Light Margarine
2 Cups	-	Whole Kernel Corn (frozen)
1 Cup	-	Heavy Cream
1 Cup	-	Half & Half Milk
1 Cup	-	Cheddar Cheese (Reduce Fat)
1 Cup	-	Water
1	-	Chicken Bouillon Cube

Preparation:

1. In medium saucepan add broccoli, margarine, water, bouillon cube, corn, cream and half and half. Simmer approx. 20 min.

2. Add cheese and simmer until thick. Add more cheese if needed.

Recommend 1 Cup Per Serving

===

BBQ SAUCE

½ Cup	-	BBQ Sauce (your choice)
3 Tbsp.	-	Ketchup
2 Tbsp.	-	Splenda Sugar Blend for Baking
1 Tsp.	-	Hot Sauce

Preparation:

1. In medium bowl combine all the above ingredients.

2. Mix well and brush on pork, chicken, turkey, or beef.

TOMATO SAUCE

1 sm.	-	Tomato
1 sm.	-	Onion (Chopped)
2 Cups	-	Water
1 Tbsp.	-	House Seasoning
3 Tbsp.	-	Tomato Paste
1 Tbsp.	-	Light Margarine
1 Tbsp.	-	Splenda Sugar Blend for Baking
1	-	Chicken Bouillon Cube

Preparation:

1. Dice onion and tomatoes in small pieces. In medium saucepan add margarine, onion, tomatoes; sauté until tender.

2. Add water, chicken bouillon cube, tomato paste, splenda sugar and house seasoning. Simmer until thick, add more water if necessary.

Recommend 1/3 Cup per serving

==

ONION GRAVY

1 Lg.	-	Onion (Chopped)
3 Tbsp.	-	Light Margarine
1 Tbsp.	-	House Seasoning
2 Tbsp.	-	Wheat Flour
2	-	Chicken Bouillon Cubes
2 Cups	-	Water

Preparation:

1. In medium saucepan or skillet, add margarine, onion and flour; sauté until onions are tender.

2. Add water, house seasoning and bouillon cubes. Stir until well blended, simmer until gravy is thick and serve.

Recommend 1/3 Cup per serving

GIBLET GRAVY

1 Pkg.	-	Chicken Gizzards
4 Cups	-	Water
3	-	Chicken Bouillon Cube
2 Cups	-	Dressing Mixture
1 Can	-	Cream Of Chicken Soup

Preparation:

1. In medium saucepan add gizzards, water and bouillon cubes; boil approx. 1 ½ hours or until gizzards are tender. Add more water if necessary.

2. Remove gizzards and cut in small pieces. Make sure there are 2 Cups of liquid in pot. Add dressing mixture, Cream Of Chicken soup and gizzards. Simmer approx. 20 min or until thick. Serve over dressing.

Recommend 1/3 Cup per serving

==

CREAM SAUCE

½	-	Red Bell Pepper
1 Cup	-	Heavy Cream
1 Tbsp.	-	Light Margarine
½ Cup	-	Chicken Broth (Low Sodium)
3 Tbsp.	-	Parmesan Cheese (in jar)

Preparation:

1. Chop pepper into small pieces. Sauté peppers and margarine until peppers are tender.

2. Add cream and chicken broth, simmer until thick. Remove from heat and add parmesan cheese. Mix well and serve.

Recommend 1/3 Cup per serving

CHEESE SAUCE

1 Cup - Half and Half Milk

1 Cup - Cheddar Cheese Reduced Fat

Preparation:

1. In medium saucepan, bring half & half to a boil; reduce heat and add cheese.

2. When cheese is completely melted pour over vegetables, potatoes, rice or pasta.

Recommend 1/3 Cup per serving

Pasta and Potatoes

SHRIMP & PASTA

½ Pkg.	-	Pasta (your choice)
1 ½ Lbs.	-	Uncooked medium shrimp (peeled and devined)
4 Tbsp.	-	Light margarine (divided)
1 Tbsp.	-	House seasoning
2 Tsp.	-	Lemon juice
½ Cup	-	Heavy Cream
1 Cube	-	Chicken Bouillon

Preparation:

1. Cook pasta according to package directions; add 2 tablespoons margarine and bouillon cube. When tender drain and set aside. (DO NOT RINSE)

2. In large skillet, sauté shrimp in 2 tablespoons margarine for approx. 4 min or until shrimp turn pink.

3. Add house seasoning, lemon juice and heavy cream to shrimp. Simmer approx 3 mins.

4. Pour shrimp mixture over pasta and serve.

Recommend 1/2 Cup per serving

===

PASTA

1 Pkg.	-	Any Pasta
1 Cube	-	Chicken Bouillon
3 Tbsp.	-	Light Margarine

Preparation:

1. Follow the directions on package and add light margarine and chicken bouillon cube.

2. When done, drain (do not rinse) and serve.

Recommend 1/3 Cup per serving

RICE

1 Cup	-	Rice
3 Tbsp.	-	Light Margarine
3 Cups	-	Water
2 Cubes	-	Chicken Bouillon

Preparation:

1. In medium saucepan combine all the above ingredients. Bring to a boil, reduce heat and cook until rice is tender.

2. Drain (do not rinse) and serve.

Recommend 1/3 Cup per serving

==

INSTANT POTATOES

1 1/3 Cups	-	Potatoes Flakes
1 1/3 Cups	-	Water
2 Tbsp.	-	Light Margarine
½ Cup	-	Heavy Cream
1 Cube	-	Chicken Bouillon
3 Tbsp.	-	Parmesan Cheese (in jar)

Preparation:

1. In medium saucepan add water, margarine and bouillon cube, bring to a boil.

2. Remove from heat, add flakes, heavy cream and mix until desired thickness. Add cheese blend and serve.

Recommend 1/3 Cup per serving

CREAM POTATOES

2 Cups	-	White Potatoes (cut up)
3 Cups	-	Water
2 Tbsp.	-	Light Margarine
½ Cup	-	Half & Half
1 Cube	-	Chicken Bouillon

Preparation:

1. Peel, wash and cut potatoes in ¼ inch squares or slices. In medium saucepan add water, margarine, bouillon cube, and potatoes. Boil until tender.

2. Remove from heat and drain. (do not rinse)

3. Mash potatoes until large lumps are gone. Add half & half and mix well.

Recommend 1/3 Cup per serving

===

POTATO STICKS

2 lg.	-	White Potatoes
1 Tbsp.	-	Low Fat Oil
1 Tbsp.	-	House Seasoning

Preparation: Preheat oven 400F

1. Peel and slice potatoes in ¼ inch slices. Cut slices in ¼ inch strips. Looks like french fries.

2. In large bowl sprinkle low fat oil and house seasoning over potatoes sticks, toss until potatoes are well coated with house seasoning.

3. Place on non-stick baking sheet and bake 400F approx. 15 min. or until tender and crisp.

Recommend 6 sticks per serving

STOVE TOP CHEESE POTATOES

2 Cups	-	White Potatoes (sliced)
1 lg.	-	Onion (sliced)
2 Tbsp.	-	Light Margarine
2/3 Cup	-	Chicken Broth (Low Sodium)
1 Cup	-	Cheddar Cheese (Reduced Fat)
		House Seasoning

Preparation:

1. Peel and slice potatoes and onion in ¼ inch slices. Sprinkle with house seasoning on both sides making sure potatoes and onions are well seasoned.

2. In large skillet, melt margarine add potatoes and top with onions. Add chicken broth cover and simmer until potatoes are tender approx. 40 min.

3. Add cheese cover and simmer until cheese has melted.

Recommend 1/3 Cup per serving

==

CORN & PASTA

2 Cups	-	Pasta (your choice)
2 Cups	-	Frozen Corn
1 Cup	-	Cheddar Cheese (Reduced Fat)
3 Tbsp.	-	Light Margarine
1 Cup	-	Half & Half Milk
1 Cube	-	Chicken Bouillon

Preparation:

1. Cook pasta according to package directions; add 2 tablespoon margarine and chicken bouillon cube. When tender drain and set aside. (Do not rinse)

2. In small saucepan combine half & half and cheese. Simmer over low heat until cheese has melted.

3. Pour noodles in casserole dish, add corn and pour cheese mixture over corn and noodles. Bake 350F approx. 30 to 40 min.

Recommend 1/2 Cup per serving

SHRIMP & RICE

1 Lb.	-	Shrimp (cooked)
½ Pkg.	-	Green Onions (chopped)
2 Cups	-	Rice (cooked)
3 Tbsp.	-	Light Margarine
½ Cup	-	Chicken Broth
1 Tbsp.	-	House Seasoning

Preparation:

1. Cook rice and set aside. Cut onions in small pieces.

2. In large skillet sauté onions and margarine until onions are tender.

3. Add cooked shrimp, house seasoning, chicken broth and cooked rice, simmer approx. 3 min. or until mixture is well heated.

Recommend 1/2 Cup per serving

===

RICE, BROCCOLI & PARMESAN CHEESE

1/4 Cup	-	Rice
1 1/4 Cup	-	Chicken Broth (low sodium)
1 Cup	-	Broccoli Florets
2 Tbsp.	-	Light Margarine
3 Tbsp.	-	Parmesan Cheese (in jar)

Preparation:

1. In medium saucepan add rice, chicken broth and margarine. Bring to boil, reduce heat and simmer until tender.

2. Add broccoli florets, toss to combine. Loosely cover and simmer 3 min.

3. Sprinkle with cheese and serve.

Recommend 1/2 Cup per serving

ORANGE SWEET POTATOES

6 sm.	-	Sweet Potatoes
2 Tbsp.	-	Light Margarine
1/2 Cup	-	Orange Juice
2 Tbsp.	-	Splenda Sugar Blend for Baking

Preparation:

1. Peel and cut potatoes in halves. In large skillet melt margarine and lay potatoes halves face down in skillet.

2. Combine orange juice and splenda mix well. Pour over potatoes halves cover and simmer approx. 20 min. or until tender turning frequently.

Recommend 2 halves per serving

===

SWEET POTATO CASSEROLE

4 Cups	-	Sweet Potatoes (cooked)
2/3 Cup	-	Water
1 Cup	-	Splenda Sugar Blend for Baking
1/2 Cup	-	Half & Half Milk
1/2 Cup	-	Light Margarine
1 Tsp.	-	Cinnamon
1/2 Tsp.	-	Nutmeg
1 Tbsp.	-	Lemon Juice
1 Tbsp.	-	Vanilla
2	-	Eggs
1/2 Cup	-	Nuts (Optional)

Preparation: Preheat oven 350F

1. Peel and cut potatoes in 1/4 inch pieces. In large pot add water and potatoes simmer until very tender.

2. Drain and pour in large mixing bowl. Add margarine and remaining ingredients. Mix by hand until well blended.

3. Pour in baking dish and bake approx. 30 to 40 min. (sprinkle with nuts).

Recommend 1/2 Cup per serving

STEWED SWEET POTATOES

2 Cups	-	Sweet Potatoes
1/2 Cup	-	Water
1/2 Cup	-	Splenda Sugar Blend for Baking
1/2 Tsp.	-	Cinnamon
2 Tbsp.	-	Light Margarine
1 Tsp.	-	Lemon Juice
1 Tsp.	-	Vanilla

Preparation:

1. Peel and cut potatoes in 1/4 inch pieces.

2. In medium saucepan combine potatoes and water cover and simmer until potatoes are tender. Drain excess water.

3. Add remaining ingredients and mix well. (Do not beat, potatoes should be lumpy)

Recommend 1/2 Cup per serving

==

FRIED SWEET POTATOES

2 lg.	-	Sweet Potatoes
1 Tbsp.	-	Low Fat Oil
4 Tbsp.	-	Light Margarine

Preparation:

1. Peel potatoes and slice 1/4 inch thick. In large skillet add low fat oil, spread over entire bottom and heat.

2. Cover the bottom of skillet with potatoes do not stack. Cook until brown on both sides and potatoes are tender.

3. Remove and repeat the process with the next batch of potatoes. Serve with 1 tablespoon of light margarine per serving.

Recommend 1/2 Cup per serving

SWEET POTATO STICKS

2 lg.	-	Sweet Potatoes
1 Tbsp.	-	Low Fat Oil
1 Tbsp.	-	Splenda Sugar Blend for Baking

Preparation: Preheat oven 400 F

1. Peel potatoes and slice in 1/4 inch slices. Cut slices in 1/4 strips. Place in large bowl.

2. Sprinkle with low fat oil and splenda sugar, toss to coat potatoes.

3. On large baking sheet spread potatoes evenly on sheet (do not stack). Bake at 400F for approx. 30 min or until potatoes are crisp. (Optional: Serve with light margarine)

Recommend 1/2 Cup per serving

===

CANDIED YAMS

3 med.	-	Sweet Potatoes
3 Tbsp.	-	Light Margarine
1/2 Cup	-	Splenda Sugar Blend for Baking
1/2 Cup	-	Water
1/4 Tsp.	-	Nutmeg
1/2 Tsp.	-	Cinnamon
1 Tsp.	-	Lemon Juice
1 Tsp.	-	Vanilla

Preparation:

1. Peel and cut potatoes in 1/4 inch pieces. In medium saucepan combine potatoes, margarine, nutmeg, cinnamon, lemon juice and vanilla.

2. Add water and sprinkle splenda sugar over the top cover and simmer until potatoes are tender approx. 20 to 25 min.

Recommend 1/2 Cup per serving

MACARONI & CHEESE

1 (8 oz.) Pkg.	-	Macaroni
1 Cube	-	Chicken Bouillon
2 Tbsp.	-	Light Margarine
2 1/2 Cups	-	Cheddar Cheese (Reduced Fat)
1 1/2 Cups	-	Half & Half Milk
2	-	Eggs (slightly beaten)

Preparation: Preheat oven 350F

1. Follow package directions for macaroni and add margarine and chicken bouillon cube. When tender, drain (do not rinse) and set aside.

2. In medium bowl combine half and half with beaten eggs, mix well.

3. Add egg mixture and 1 1/2 Cups of cheese to macaroni and blend well. Pour in baking dish and sprinkle remaining cheese over top.

4. Cover and bake at 350 for 35 min. Uncover turn oven to broil and brown top. Remove and serve.

Recommend 1/2 Cup per serving

===

MACARONI SALAD

1 Cup	-	Macaroni
1 Cube	-	Chicken Bouillon
2 Tbsp.	-	Light Margarine
3 Tbsp.	-	Light Mayonnaise
2 Tbsp.	-	Pickle Relish
1/4	-	Onion (chopped) Optional
2	-	Eggs (boiled)

Preparation:

1. Follow package directions for macaroni and add margarine and Chicken bouillon cube. When tender drain (do not rinse) and set aside. Boil eggs in small pot.

2. Cut up eggs and onion, add all the above ingredients including macaroni in large bowl, mix until well coated. Serve warm or cold.

Recommend 1/2 Cup per serving

Vegetables

GREEN BEANS & RADISH

1 (16) Pkg.	-	Frozen Green Beans
1 Cup	-	Radish (thinly sliced)
1/2	-	Onion (thinly sliced)
1/3 Cup	-	Chicken Broth
3 Tbsp.	-	Light Margarine
1/2 Tsp.	-	Splenda Sugar Blend for Baking
1/3 Cup	-	Italian Low Fat Dressing

Preparation:

1. In large skillet sauté margarine, green beans and onions. When beans and onions are well coated with margarine add chicken broth, cover and steam until beans are tender.

2. Add radish, splenda sugar and Italian dressing. Toss making sure all beans and radishes are completely coated with dressing.

Recommend 1/2 Cup per serving

===

GREEN BEANS

1 (16 oz.) Pkg.	-	Frozen Green Beans
2 Tbsp.	-	Light Margarine
2 Tsp.	-	Splenda Sugar Blend for Baking
1 Tbsp.	-	House Seasoning
1 Cup	-	Water
1/2	-	Onion (sliced)
1 Cube	-	Chicken Bouillon

Preparation:

1. Cut onion in small slices. In medium saucepan add remaining ingredients.

2. Cover and boil over medium heat approx. 35 min. or until beans are tender.

Recommend 1/2 Cup per serving

SAUTED GREEN BEANS

1 (16 oz.) Pkg.	-	Frozen Green Beans
3 Tbsp.	-	Light Margarine
1/2	-	Onion (sliced)
2 Tsp.	-	Splenda Sugar Blend for Baking
1 Tbsp.	-	House Seasoning

Preparation:

1. In large skillet melt margarine. Add beans, onion, house seasoning and splenda.

2. Sauté until beans are tender approx. 20 min.

Recommend 1/2 Cup per serving

===

GREEN BEANS & TOMATOES

1 (16 oz.) Pkg.	-	Frozen Green Beans
1 lg.	-	Tomato
2 Tbsp.	-	Light Margarine
2 Tsp.	-	Splenda Sugar Blend for Baking
1 Tbsp.	-	House Seasoning
1 Cup	-	Water
1/2	-	Onion (chopped)
1 Cube	-	Chicken Bouillon

Preparation:

1. Cut onion in small pieces, cut tomato in 1/4 inch pieces.

2. In medium saucepan add all ingredients. Cover and bring to boil, reduce heat and simmer approx. 35 min. or until beans are tender.

Recommend 1/2 Cup per serving

BUTTER BEANS & ORKA

1 (16 oz.) Pkg.	-	Frozen Butter Beans
1 (8 oz.) Pkg.	-	Frozen Orka
2 Tbsp.	-	Light Margarine
2 Tsp.	-	Splenda Sugar Blend for Baking
1/2	-	Onion (sliced)
2 Cups	-	Water
1 Cube	-	Chicken Bouillon
1 Tbsp	-	House Seasoning

Preparation:

1. In medium saucepan cut up onion and add beans, house seasoning, margarine, water and bouillon cube. Add orka on top of beans and sprinkle with splenda.

2. Bring to a boil, reduce heat cover and simmer approx. 35 to 40 min. or until beans are tender.

Recommend 1/2 Cup per serving

==

GREEN BEANS & CORN

1 (16 oz.) Pkg.	-	Frozen Green Beans
1 Cup	-	Frozen Whole Kernel Corn
3 Tbsp.	-	Light Margarine
1/2	-	Onion (sliced)
1 Cup	-	Water
2 Tsp.	-	Splenda Sugar Blend for Baking
1 Tbsp.	-	House Seasoning
1 Cube	-	Chicken Bouillon

Preparation:

1. Cut onion in small slices. In medium saucepan add remaining ingredients.

2. Cover and simmer over medium heat for approx. 35 min. or until beans are tender.

Recommend 1/2 Cup per serving

MIX VEGETABLES

1 (16 oz.) Pkg.	-	Mix Vegetables (any kind)
2 Tbsp.	-	Light Margarine
2 Tsp.	-	Splenda Sugar Blend for Baking
1 Tbsp.	-	House Seasoning
1/2 Cup	-	Chicken Broth (low sodium)

Preparation:

1. In medium saucepan combine margarine, mix vegetables, chicken broth, house seasoning and splenda sugar.

2. Cook over medium heat until vegetables are tender. Stirring occasionally. (Read instructions on bag for cooking time).

Recommend 1/2 Cup per serving

==

PURPLE HULL PEAS

1 (16 oz.) Pkg.	-	Frozen Purple Hull Peas
1/2	-	Onion (chopped)
2 Tbsp.	-	Light Margarine
1 Tbsp.	-	House Seasoning
2 Tsp.	-	Splenda Sugar Blend for Baking
2 1/2 Cups	-	Water
1 Cube	-	Chicken Bouillon

Preparation:

1. In medium saucepan, add all the above ingredients. Cover and bring to a boil.

2. Reduce heat and simmer until peas are soft approx. 40 to 45 min. (Add additional water if necessary)

Recommend 1/2 Cups per serving

BLACKEYED PEAS

1 (16 oz.) Pkg.	-	Frozen Black-eyed Peas
1/2	-	Onion (chopped)
2 Tbsp.	-	Light Margarine
1 Tbsp.	-	House Seasoning
2 Tsp.	-	Splenda Sugar Blend for Baking
2 1/2 Cup	-	Water
1 Cube	-	Chicken Bouillon

Preparation:

1. In medium saucepan add all the above ingredients. Cover and bring to a boil.

2. Reduce heat and simmer until peas are tender approx. 40 to 45 min. (Add additional water if necessary)

Recommend 1/2 Cup per serving

===

TRUNIP GREENS

1 (16 oz.) Pkg.	-	Frozen Turnip Greens
1 Cube	-	Chicken Bouillon
2 Tbsp.	-	Light Margarine
2 Tsp.	-	Splenda Sugar Blend for Baking
1/2	-	Onion (sliced)
1 1/2 Cup	-	Water

Preparation:

1. Cut onion into small pieces. Combine all ingredients in medium saucepan.

2. Bring to a boil, reduce heat cover and simmer approx. 30 to 40 min.

Recommend 1/2 Cup per serving

COLLARD GREENS

1 (16 oz.) Pkg.	-	Frozen Collard Greens
1 Cube	-	Chicken Bouillon
2 Tbsp.	-	Light Margarine
2 Tsp.	-	Splenda Sugar Blend for Baking
1/2	-	Onion (chopped)
1 1/2 Cup	-	Water

Preparation:

1. Cut onion into small pieces. Combine all ingredients into medium saucepan.

2. Bring to a boil, reduce heat cover and simmer approx. 30 to 40 min.

Recommend 1/2 Cup per serving

==

SMOTHERED CABBAGE

1	-	Head Cabbage (cut-up)
1 Cube	-	Chicken Bouillon
3 Tbsp.	-	Light Margarine
1 Tbsp.	-	House Seasoning
2 Tsp.	-	Splenda Sugar Blend for Baking
1 Cup	-	Water

Preparation:

1. Cut up cabbage and wash. In large pot add margarine and let melt. Add water, bouillon cube, cabbage, house seasoning and splenda.

2. Cover and steam, stirring occasionally until cabbage are tender. (do not over cook)

Recommend 1/2 Cup per serving

MUSTARD GREENS

1 (16 oz.) Pkg.	-	Frozen Mustard Greens
1 Cube	-	Chicken Bouillon
2 Tbsp.	-	Light Margarine
2 Tsp.	-	Splenda Sugar Blend for Baking
1/2	-	Onion (chopped)
1 1/2 Cup	-	Water

Preparation:

1. Cut onion into small pieces. Combine all ingredients in medium saucepan.

2. Bring to a boil, reduce heat cover and simmer approx. 30 to 40 min.

Recommend 1/2 Cup per serving

===

ASPARAGUS

1 Bunch	-	Fresh Asparagus
3 Tbsp.	-	Light Margarine (melted)
1 Tsp.	-	Splenda Sugar Blend for Baking
4	-	Green Onions (chopped)
1/3 Cup	-	Chicken Broth (low sodium)

Preparation:

1. Wash and trim asparagus. Spray shallow baking dish with cooking spray and add asparagus and green onions.

2. Pour melted margarine over onions and sprinkle with splenda. Place in oven and bake approx. 15 min. or until lightly brown.

Recommend 1/2 Cup per serving

SWEET PEAS

1 (16 oz.) Pkg.	-	Frozen Sweet Peas
2 Tbsp.	-	Light Margarine
2 Tsp.	-	Splenda Sugar Blend for Baking
1/2 Cup	-	Chicken Broth

Preparation:

1. In medium saucepan combine all the above ingredients.

2. Cover and simmer until peas are tender approx. 20 min.

Recommend 1/2 Cup per serving

===

BROCCOLI & CHEESE

1 (16 oz.) Pkg.	-	Frozen Broccoli
1/2 Cup	-	Chicken Broth (Low sodium)
1/2 Cup	-	Heavy Cream
1 Cup	-	Cheddar Cheese (Reduced Fat)
2 Tbsp.	-	Light Margarine

Preparation:

1. Combine broccoli, margarine and chicken broth in medium skillet. Cover and simmer until broccoli is tender.

2. Drain off excess liquid. Add heavy cream and sprinkle cheese over broccoli. Heat until cheese has melted. Toss to coat broccoli pieces.

Recommend 1/2 Cup per serving

SAUTED BROCCOLI

1 (16 oz.) Pkg.	-	Frozen Broccoli
1/2 Cup	-	Chicken Broth
2 Tbsp.	-	Light Margarine
2 Tsp.	-	Splenda Sugar Blend for Baking

Preparation:

1. In large skillet heat margarine. Add broccoli and sauté for approx. 2 min. Add chicken broth and splenda.

2. Sauté broccoli until tender.

Recommend 1/2 Cup per serving

===

CORN ON COB

6 Ears	-	Frozen or Fresh Corn
3 Tbsp.	-	Light Margarine
2 Tbsp.	-	Splenda Sugar Blend for Baking

Preparation:

1. In large saucepan add all the above ingredients.

2. Cover the corn with water and boil over medium heat until corn is tender approx. 40 min.

Recommend 1 small ear or 1/2 of large ear per serving

===

WHOLE KERNEL CORN

1 (16 oz.) Pkg.	-	Frozen Kernel Corn
1/2 Cup	-	Heavy Cream
3 Tbsp.	-	Light Margarine
2 Tsp.	-	Splenda Sugar Blend for Baking

Preparation:

1. In medium saucepan add all ingredients.

2. Cover and bring to boil, reduce heat and simmer until corn is tender approx. 25 min.

Recommend 1/2 Cup per serving

GLAZED CARROTS

1 (16 oz.) Pkg.	-	Frozen Cut Carrots
2 Tbsp.	-	Light Margarine
2 Tsp.	-	Splenda Sugar Blend for Baking
1/3 Cup	-	Chicken Broth

Preparation:

1. In medium skillet or saucepan combine carrots and chicken broth. Cover and steam until carrots are tender. (Drain)

2. Sprinkle with splenda sugar and margarine. Sauté until carrots are glazed with margarine and splenda.

Recommend 1/2 Cup per serving

===

WHOLE CARROTS

1 (16 oz.) Pkg.	-	Frozen Whole Carrots
1/2 Cup	-	Chicken Broth
2 Tsp.	-	Splenda Sugar Blend for Baking
2 Tbsp.	-	Light Margarine

Preparation:

1. In a medium saucepan combine all the above ingredients.

2. Bring to a boil, reduce heat and simmer approx. 20 to 25 min. or until carrots are tender.

Recommend 1/2 Cup per serving

WHOLE ORKA

1 (16 oz.) Pkg.	-	Frozen Orka
2 Tsp.	-	Splenda Sugar Blend for Baking
2 Tbsp.	-	Light Margarine
1 Cup	-	Water
1 Cube	-	Chicken Bouillon

Preparation:

1. In medium saucepan combine orka, margarine, water and chicken bouillon cube. Sprinkle splenda sugar over top of orka.

2. Cover and boil over low heat until orka is tender, approx. 20 to 30 min.

Recommend 1/2 Cup per serving

===

ORKA & TOMATOES

1 (16 oz.) Pkg.	-	Frozen Cut Orka
1 lg.	-	Tomato (cut-up)
1/2 Cup	-	Chicken Broth
3 Tbsp.	-	Light Margarine
2 Tsp.	-	House Seasoning
2 Tsp.	-	Splenda Sugar Blend for Baking

Preparation:

1. Dice tomato into small pieces. In medium skillet add all the above ingredients.

2. Cover and simmer until orka is very tender stirring occasionally approx. 25 min.

3. Add additional chicken broth if necessary.

Recommend 1/2 Cup per serving

SQUASH

1 (16 oz.) Pkg.	-	Frozen cut Squash
1 sm.	-	Onion (sliced)
1/2 Cup	-	Chicken Broth
2 Tbsp.	-	Light Margarine
1 Tbsp.	-	House Seasoning
2 Tsp.	-	Splenda Sugar Blend for Baking

Preparation:

1. Slice onion. In medium skillet add all the above ingredients. Cover and simmer approx. 15 min.

2. Uncover and simmer an additional 15 min. stirring occasionally.

3. Add additional chicken broth if needed.

Recommend 1/2 Cup per serving

==

GRILLED SQUASH

2 med.	-	Squash (1/4 inch slices)
1 Tbsp.	-	House Seasoning
2 Tsp.	-	Splenda Sugar Blend for Baking

Preparation:

1. Cut squash in 1/4 inch slices. In small bowl combine splenda and house seasoning. Sprinkle squash on both sides.

2. Spray grill with cooking spray and place squash on grill. Turn squash every 5 min.

3. When tender remove and serve.

Recommend 1/2 Cup per serving

GOURMET SQUASH

3	-	Yellow Squash (cut in halves)
2/3 Cup	-	Diced Celery
1 1/2 Cups	-	Diced Apples
3 Tbsp.	-	Light Margarine
1 Cup	-	Cheddar Cheese (Reduced Fat)
1/2 Cup	-	Chicken Broth (Low Sodium)

Preparation: Preheat oven 400F

1. Cut squash in half and remove seeds. Place cut side face down on baking pan. Add half of chicken broth. Bake for approx. 25 min.

2. Dice apples and celery and sauté in light margarine for approx. 5 min. add cheese and remove from heat.

3. Turn squash halves face up and fill with apple mixture. Add remaining chicken broth.

4. Bake 10 or 15 min. or until squash are tender.

Recommend 1 baked half per serving

===

CARROT-APPLE CASSEROLE

2 Cups	-	Frozen Sliced Carrots
2 Cups	-	Frozen Apples
1 Tbsp.	-	Lemon Juice
1 Tbsp.	-	Splenda Sugar Blend for Baking
2 Tbsp.	-	Light Margarine
1/2 Cup	-	Water

Preparation: Preheat oven 350F

1. Place apples and carrots in a 1 quart baking dish. Sprinkle with lemon juice, water and splenda.

2. Add margarine and mix well making sure apples and carrots are well coated.

3. Bake approx. 35 to 40 min. or until carrots are tender.

Recommend 1/2 Cup per serving

SAUTED CAULIFLOWER

2 Cups	-	Cauliflower (sliced)
1 Cup	-	Onion (thinly sliced)
1 Cup	-	Celery (thinly sliced)
1/2 Cup	-	Chicken Broth (Low sodium)
3 Tbsp.	-	Light Margarine
2 Tsp.	-	Splenda Sugar Blend for Baking
2 Tsp.	-	House Seasoning

Preparation:

1. Cut up all vegetables. Melt margarine in large skillet. Add cauliflower, celery, onion, splenda and house seasoning. Mix well.

2. Place over low heat and add chicken broth heat approx. 3 min. Turn heat to medium high and cook quickly until vegetables are barely tender and crisp. Approx. 7 to 8 min. Turn over constantly.

Recommend 1/2 Cup per serving

ZUCCHINI CASSEROLE

4 Cups	-	Zucchini (Sliced)
1 Lb.	-	Ground Turkey
1 Cup	-	Cheddar Cheese (Reduced Fat)
1 Cup	-	Parmesan Cheese
1 Cup	-	Half & Half Milk
1 sm.	-	Onion (Chopped)
1 Tbsp.	-	House Seasoning
2	-	Eggs (Slightly Beaten)

Preparation: Preheat Oven 350F

1. Slice Zucchini, place in large saucepan add 1/2 Cup water and steam until tender approx. 15 min.

2. In large skillet add ground turkey, onion and house seasoning cook until brown.

3. Beat eggs add milk and blend well.

4. In large bowl, add milk and egg mixture; add 1/2 Cup of cheddar cheese and parmesan cheese mix well.

5. In a casserole dish add zucchini and ground turkey, pour milk and cheese mixture over turkey. Sprinkle top with remaining cheese.

6. Cover and bake approx. 40 min. Remove cover half way through to form a cheese crust.

Recommend 1/2 Cup per serving

Meats

STUFFED CHICKEN BREAST

4	-	Chicken Breast
1/2 Cup	-	Onion (diced)
1/2 Cup	-	Celery (diced)
1 Cup	-	Chicken Broth (Low sodium)
1/2 Cup	-	Cheddar Cheese (Reduced Fat)
2 Tsp.	-	Splenda Sugar Blend for Baking
		House Seasoning

Preparation:

1. Wash and remove skin from breast. Make a slit in fat end, all the way down the breast (Do not cut all the way through.) Make a pocket.

2. Season breast inside and outside with house seasoning. Make sure breast are well seasoned.

3. In a small bowl combine onion, celery, splenda sugar and cheese mix well.

4. Stuff each breast with cheese mixture and close with wooden toothpick.

5. Heat margarine in large skillet. Brown breast on both sides over medium heat. Add chicken broth cover and simmer over low heat turning every 15 min.

6. After 30 min. uncover and cook additional 15 min. Remove toothpicks and serve with remaining juice over chicken breast.

Recommend 1/2 breast per serving
Approx. 3 oz.

BAKED CHICKEN

1 - Chicken (cut-up)

House Seasoning

Preparation:

1. Wash and remove skin from chicken. Sprinkle house seasoning generously on both sides of chicken.

2. Place in foil and bake approx. 45 to 50 min. Uncover turn oven to broil and brown on both sides.

3. Remove and serve.

Recommend 3 oz. per serving

==

BAKED CHICKEN WINGS

1 Pkg. - Chicken Wings

House Seasoning

Preparation:

1. Wash and sprinkle wings with house seasoning, making sure wings are well coated with seasoning.

2. Place in foil and bake approx. 40 to 45 min. Uncover turn oven to broil and brown wings on both sides.

Recommend 3 oz. per serving

CHICKEN & GRAVY

1 - Chicken (Cut up) or chicken parts
House Seasoning

GRAVY

2 Tbsp.	-	Light Margarine
2 Tbsp.	-	Wheat Flour
1 Tbsp.	-	House Seasoning
1 sm.	-	Onion (Chopped)
2	-	Chicken Bouillon Cubes
2 Cups	-	Water

Preparation: Preheat oven 350F

1. Cut up, wash and season chicken with house seasoning.

2. Wrap in foil and place in oven approx. 40 min. Uncover, turn oven to broil and brown on both sides.

3. Sauté margarine, flour and onions until onions are tender. Add water, chicken bouillon cubes and 1 Tbsp. house seasoning. Bring to boil reduce heat.

4. Add chicken to gravy and simmer approx. 15 min or until gravy is thick.

5. Serve with rice, potatoes or pasta.

Recommend 1 piece of chicken and 3 Tbsp. gravy.

CHICKEN GIZZARDS

1 Pkg.	-	Chicken Gizzards
1 Tbsp.	-	House Seasoning
3 Tbsp.	-	Light Margarine
1 sm.	-	Onion (Chopped)
1 Cup	-	Cheddar Cheese (Reduced Fat)
1/2 Cup	-	Heavy Cream
3 Cups	-	Water
2	-	Chicken Bouillon Cubes

Preparation:

1. Wash and clean gizzards. In medium saucepan add gizzards, onion, house seasoning, margarine, water and bouillon cubes.

2. Bring to boil, reduce heat and boil approx 1 to 1 1/2 hrs. or until gizzards are tender.

3. Add heavy cream and cheese to gizzards and simmer until sauce is thick.

Recommend 1/2 Cup per serving

===

STOVE TOP CHICKEN

1	-	Chicken (Cut up) or parts
1/2 Cup	-	Chicken Broth (Low Sodium)
1 Tbsp.	-	Oil (Low Fat)
		House Seasoning

Preparation:

1. Preheat large skillet with low fat oil, spread oil until bottom of skillet is covered.

2. Wash and remove skin, sprinkle with house seasoning making sure chicken is well seasoned on both sides.

3. Add chicken to hot oil and brown on both sides.

4. When chicken is brown on both sides add chicken broth cover and simmer approx. 45 min. turning every 15 min.

5. Serve liquid over chicken.

Recommend 3 oz. per serving

TOSS CHICKEN

1 Lb.	-	Chicken Cutlets
1 Tbsp.	-	Cornstarch
1 Tbsp.	-	Low Fat Oil
1/2	-	Onion (Chopped)
1 Tbsp.	-	Minced Garlic
1 Tbsp.	-	House Seasoning
2 Tbsp.	-	Orange Juice
1 Tsp.	-	Splenda Sugar Blend for baking

Preparation:

1. Mix cornstarch, and house seasoning blend well. Toss chicken in cornstarch mixture.

2. Add oil to large skillet or wok on medium heat. When oil is hot add toss chicken to skillet and stir until chicken is brown, remove from skillet.

3. Add onions and garlic and fry for approx. 1 min. Mix orange juice and splenda sugar and blend well.

4. Return chicken to skillet and add orange juice and cook approx. 10 min. stirring occasionally.

5. Remove and serve.

Recommend 1/2 Cup per serving
Approx. 3 oz.

CHICKEN STIR FRY

1 lg.	-	Chicken Breast
1 (16 oz. Pkg.)	-	Stir Fry Vegetables (any brand)
4 Tbsp.	-	Light Margarine
1/2 Cup	-	Chicken Broth (Low Sodium)
1 Tbsp.	-	House Seasoning
2 Tsp.	-	Splenda Sugar Blend for Baking

Preparation:

1. Cut chicken breast into very small pieces. Sprinkle small pieces with house seasoning toss to blend well.

2. In large skillet add margarine and chicken. Sauté until chicken is no longer pink.

3. Add stir fry vegetables, chicken broth and sprinkle splenda sugar over top of vegetables.

4. Sauté until vegetables are completely cooked. Approx. 20 min.

Recommend 1/2 Cup per serving

Approx. 3 oz.

==

BBQ CHICKEN

1	-	Chicken (cut up)
		House Seasoning
		BBQ Sauce

Preparation:

1. Sprinkle house seasoning on both sides. Make sure chicken is well seasoned.

2. OVEN - Wrap chicken in foil and bake in 350F oven for approx. 45 min. Uncover and lightly brush with BBQ sauce on both sides. Turn oven to broil and bake chicken approx. 2 min. on each side. Remove and brush with remaining sauce.

3. GRILL - Place seasoned chicken on grill until chicken is tender. Lightly brush chicken with BBQ sauce on both sides and grill an additional 15 min. Remove and brush with remaining sauce.

Recommend 3 oz. per serving

CHICKEN SKILLET DINNER

2	-	Chicken Breast (Cut up)
1 Cup	-	Carrots sliced
1	-	Zucchini (Thinly sliced)
1/2 Cup	-	Onion (Chopped)
1 Cup	-	Chicken Broth (Low Sodium)
1 Cup	-	Cheddar Cheese (Reduced Fat)
1 Tbsp.	-	House Seasoning

Preparation:

1. Heat large skillet over medium heat. Sprinkle chicken with house seasoning making sure chicken is well covered.

2. Add chicken to hot skillet and stir fry until chicken is no longer pink. Remove chicken from skillet.

3. Add zucchini and carrots and stir fry approx. 5 min. or until tender.

4. Add chicken to vegetables mixture, chicken broth and 1/2 Cup of cheese. Let simmer until thick.

5. Sprinkle remaining cheese on top of chicken and serve.

Recommend 1/2 Cup per serving
Approx. 3 oz.

LEMON & GARLIC GRILL CHICKEN

1	-	Chicken (skin removed & cut up)
2 Tsp.	-	Minced Garlic
1/2 Cup	-	Lemon Juice
2 Tbsp.	-	House Seasoning
1/4 Cup	-	Low Fat Oil

Preparation:

1. Cut up chicken and remove skin.

2. Combine all the above ingredients.

3. Place chicken and marinate in large zip lock plastic bag. Make sure all pieces are covered.

4. Refrigerate 4 to 6 hours.

5. Remove chicken from marinate and place on hot grill. Use remaining marinate for basting.

Recommend 3 oz. Per serving

ROASTED CHICKEN

1 - Whole Chicken

1 - Whole Lemon

House Seasoning

Preparation: Preheat oven 350F

1. Remove giblet and neck from chicken. Wash and remove any excess fat.

2. Sprinkle house seasoning all over entire chicken making sure chicken is well covered with seasoning.

3. Place whole lemon inside cavity of chicken.

4. Place chicken on baking rack with (breast side down).

5. Bake for 1 hour, turning chicken so breast side is up and bake an additional 30 min.

Recommend 3 oz. Per serving

==

ROASTED CORNISH HEN

1 - Whole Cornish Hen

1 - Whole Lemon

House Seasoning

Preparation: Preheat oven 350F

1. Remove giblet and neck from Cornish hen. Wash and remove any excess fat.

2. Sprinkle house seasoning all over entire Cornish hen making sure Cornish hen is well covered with seasoning.

3. Place whole lemon inside cavity of Cornish hen.

4. Place Cornish hen on baking rack with (breast side down).

5. Bake for 30 min., turn Cornish hen so breast side is up and bake an additional 30 min.

Recommend 3 oz. Per serving

BBQ PORK CHOPS

6 - Pork chops
House seasoning
BBQ Sauce

Preparation:

1. Sprinkle house seasoning on both sides. Make sure chops are well seasoned.

2. OVEN - Wrap chops in foil and bake in 350F oven for approx. 45 min. Uncover and lightly brush with BBQ sauce on both sides. Turn oven to broil and bake chops approx. 2 min on each side. Remove and brush with remaining sauce.

3. GRILL - Place seasoned chops on grill until chops are tender. Lightly brush chops with BBQ sauce on both sides and grill an additional 15 min. Remove and brush with remaining sauce.

Recommend 3 oz. Per serving

==

ORANGE PORK CHOPS & ONIONS

4	-	Pork Chops
1 lg.	-	Onion (sliced)
1 Tsp.	-	Splenda Sugar Blend for Baking
1/2 Cup	-	Orange Juice
1 Tbsp.	-	Low Fat Oil
		House Seasoning

Preparation:

1. Sprinkle chops with house seasoning on both sides. Make sure chops are well seasoned.

2. In large skillet heat oil, when hot add chops and brown on both sides.

3. In small bowl, combine orange juice and splenda, mix well. Add sliced onions and orange juice mixture cover and simmer 40 to 45 min or until chops are tender.

4. Serve with onions on top of chops.

Recommend 3 oz. per serving

STOVE TOP PORK CHOPS

4	-	Pork Chops
1/2 Cup	-	Chicken Broth (Low Sodium)
1 Tbsp.	-	Low Fat Oil
		House Seasoning

Preparation:

1. Preheat large skillet with oil, spread oil until bottom of skillet is covered. Sprinkle chops with house seasoning making sure chops are seasoned on both sides.

2. Add chops to hot oil and brown on both sides.

3. When brown, add chicken broth and simmer approx. 40 to 45 min. turning every 15 min. Serve with liquid over chops.

Recommend 3 oz. per serving

==

PORK CHOPS DELIGHT

4	-	Pork Chops
1 lg.	-	Tomato
1 lg.	-	Red Bell Pepper
1 lg.	-	Onion
1 Tbsp.	-	Low Fat Oil
1/2 Cup	-	Chicken Broth (Low Sodium)
		House Seasoning

Preparation:

1. Heat oil in large skillet. Sprinkle chops with house seasoning on both sides. Place in skillet and brown.

2. Cut pepper, tomato and onion in thick slices. Sprinkle with house seasoning and stack a slice of pepper, onion and tomatoes on top of each chop.

3. Add chicken broth, cover and simmer 30 to 40 min or until chops are tender. Dip liquid over entire stack before serving.

Recommend 3 oz. per serving

BAKED PORK CHOPS

4 - Pork Chops
House Seasoning

Preparation:

1. Sprinkle house seasoning generously on both sides of pork chops. Place in foil, cover and bake approx. 35 to 40 min. or until chops are tender.

2. Uncover turn oven to broil and brown on both sides. Remove & serve.

Recommend 3 oz. per servings

===

STUFFED PORK CHOPS

4	-	Pork Chops 1/2 inch thick
1/2 Cup	-	Onion (diced)
1/2 Cup	-	Celery (diced)
1 Cup	-	Chicken Broth (Low Sodium)
1/2 Cup	-	Cheddar Cheese (Reduced Fat)
2 Tsp.	-	Splenda Sugar Blend for Baking
		House Seasoning

Preparation:

1. Make a slit in fat end all the way down chops making a pocket. (Do not cut all the way through)

2. Season chops inside and outside with house seasoning. Make sure chops are well seasoned.

3. In a small bowl combine onion, celery, splenda sugar and cheese mix well.

4. Stuff each chop with cheese mixture and close with wooden toothpick.

5. Heat margarine in large skillet. Brown chops on both sides over medium heat. Add chicken broth cover and simmer over low heat turning every 15 min.

6. After 30 min. uncover and cook additional 15 min. Remove toothpicks and serve with remaining juice over pork chops.

Recommend 3 oz. Per serving

BBQ RIBS

1 slab - Ribs
House Seasoning
BBQ Sauce

Preparation:

1. Sprinkle house seasoning on both sides. Make sure ribs are well seasoned.

2. OVEN - Wrap ribs in foil and bake in 350F oven for approx. 1 hr. and 45 min. Uncover and lightly brush with BBQ sauce on both sides. Turn oven to broil and bake ribs approx. 2 min on each side. Remove and brush with remaining sauce.

2. GRILL - Place seasoned ribs on grill until ribs are tender. Lightly brush chops with BBQ sauce on both sides and grill an additional 15 min. Remove and brush with remaining sauce.

Recommend 3 oz. Per serving

==

TURKEY MEATLOAF

1 Lb.	-	Ground Turkey
1 sm.	-	Onion (chopped)
2 Tbsp.	-	Wheat Flour
4 Tbsp.	-	BBQ Sauce (divided)
2 Tbsp.	-	House Seasoning
1	-	Egg

Preparation: Preheat oven 350F

1. In large bowl, add chopped onions, ground turkey, house seasoning, eggs, wheat flour and 2 tablespoons BBQ sauce. Mix well with hands.

2. Shape in a meatloaf form, top with remaining BBQ sauce and bake approx. 40 to 50 min.

Recommend 3 oz. per serving

TURKEY MEATBALLS

1 Lb.	-	Ground Turkey
1 sm.	-	Onion (chopped)
2 Tbsp.	-	Wheat Flour
2 Tbsp.	-	BBQ Sauce
2 Tbsp.	-	House Seasoning
1	-	Egg

Preparation: Preheat oven 350F

1. Combine all the above ingredients in large bowl. Mix well with hands.

2. Form the size meatballs you desire.

3. Place on non-stick baking sheet and bake approx. 20 to 25 min. Prepare tomato sauce recipe and add to meatballs.

Recommend 3 oz. per serving

===

STUFFED TURKEY BURGERS

1 Lb.	-	Ground Turkey
1	-	Onion (chopped)
2 Tbsp.	-	Wheat Flour
2 Tbsp.	-	BBQ Sauce
2 Tbsp.	-	House Seasoning
1	-	Egg
1/2 Cup	-	Mozzarella & Parmesan Cheese

Preparation: Preheat oven 350F

1. In large bowl, add 1/2 chopped onion, ground turkey, house seasoning, egg and BBQ sauce. Mix well with hands.

2. In small bowl combine cheese and remaining onion, toss to combine.

3. Make one thin burger, fill center with cheese mixture, make another thin burger place on top of cheese. Close ends of burger tightly. Make sure cheese does not leak.

4. Place burgers on non-stick baking pan. Bake approx. 25 to 30 min.

Recommend 3 oz. Per serving

SHORT RIBS

3 Lbs.	-	Short Ribs
1 Tbsp.	-	Low Fat Oil
1 lg.	-	Onion (sliced)
2	-	Chicken Bouillon Cubes
2 Cups	-	Water
		House Seasoning

Preparation:

1. Remove excess fat from ribs. Sprinkle ribs with house seasoning. Make sure ribs are well covered with seasoning.

2. Heat large skillet with oil, add ribs and brown on both sides approx. 3 min. on each side.

3. Remove ribs from skillet. Add onions and sauté until tender.

4. Add water, bouillon cube and return ribs to skillet. Bring to boil reduce heat and simmer approx. 1 1/2 hours or until ribs are tender. Add more water if needed.

Recommend 3 oz. Per serving

STOVE TOP STEAK

2	-	Steaks (your choice)
1/2 Cup	-	Beef Broth (Low sodium)
1 Tbsp.	-	Low Fat Oil
		House Seasoning

Preparation:

1. Preheat large skillet with oil. Sprinkle steaks with house seasoning on both sides. Make sure steaks are well seasoned.

2. Add steaks to hot oil and brown on both sides. Reduce heat add beef broth cover and simmer approx. 20 to 25 min. or until your desired tenderness.

3. Serve liquid over steak.

Recommend 3 oz. per serving

===

BAKED FISH

4	-	Fish Fillets (your choice)
1 Tbsp.	-	Low Fat Oil
1 Tbsp.	-	Lemon Juice
		House Seasoning

Preparation: Preheat oven 350F

1. Pour oil in pan, spread over entire bottom. Season fillets with house seasoning on both sides.

2. Bake fish until flakes with fork. Sprinkle with lemon juice and serve.

Recommend 3 oz. per serving.

PEPPER & STEAK SALAD

1	-	Steak (any kind)
1/2	-	Red bell pepper (sliced)
1/2	-	Green bell pepper (sliced)
1/2	-	Yellow bell pepper (sliced)
1/2	-	Onion (sliced)
1/2 Cup	-	Cheese cheddar
2 Tbsp		House seasoning
1 Tsp.	-	Light margarine
1/2 Cup	-	Beef broth (low sodium)

Preparation:

1. Cut steak in small strips.

2. Add steak strips and broth in large skillet and simmer until steak is tender.

3. Drain excess broth and add margarine, peppers, onion and house seasoning.

4. Sauté until peppers and onion are tender.

5. On large plate, tear lettuce apart and add cheese on top.

6. Dip steak and peppers over lettuce and cheese mixture and serve.

7. OPTIONAL (Use any light dressing)

Recommend 3 oz. Per serving

STEAK & GRAVY

1	-	Round Steak
1 Cup	-	Beef Broth (Low Sodium)
1 Tbsp.	-	Low Fat Oil
1/2	-	Onion (sliced)
1/2 Cup	-	Heavy Cream
1 Cup	-	Cheddar Cheese (Reduced Fat)
1 Cup	-	Water
		House Seasoning

Preparation:

1. Preheat large skillet with low fat oil.

2. Cut steak into strips and season well with house seasoning.

3. Add steak to hot skillet and brown on both sides. Cook until all liquid has evaporated.

4. Add onion, beef broth and water cover and simmer until meat is tender approx. 45 min.

5. Add cream and cheese, simmer until gravy is thick.

6. Serve over potatoes, rice or pasta.

Recommend 3 oz. Per serving

❧❧

Desserts

❧❧

POUND CAKE

2 Sticks	-	Land O Lakes (light butter) soften
1 2/3 Cups	-	Splenda Sugar Blend for Baking
2 1/2 Cups	-	Swans Down Cake Flour
1 Tbsp.	-	Baking Powder
1/4 Tsp.	-	Baking Soda
1 Cup	-	Fat Free Milk
1 Tbsp.	-	Vanilla Extract
6	-	Egg Yolks

Preparation: Preheat oven 350F

1. In mixing bowl combine splenda sugar, cake flour, baking powder and baking soda; mix with large spoon until well blended.

2. Cut soft butter into chunks, add to flour mixture. Mix at medium speed until mixture is crumbly; approx. 1 min.

3. Pour 1/4 Cup of milk into flour mixture; mix at low speed approx. 30 sec. Scrap sides and add remaining milk, egg yolks, and vanilla.

4. Mix on HIGH speed for 1 1/2 mins. Spray pound cake pan with (cooking spray with flour) and pour batter evenly around pan. Shake to even batter out.

5. Bake at 350F for 1 hour or until toothpick comes out clean.

Recommend 1 medium slice per serving

PECAN PIE

1 Cup	-	Karo Syrup Dark
6	-	Eggs (slightly beaten)
1 Cup	-	Splenda sugar blend for baking
4 Tbsp.	-	Melted Light Butter
1 Tbsp.	-	Vanilla
2 1/2 Cups	-	Pecans
2 (9")	-	Unbaked pie crust

Preparation: Preheat oven 350F

1. Combine first 5 (five) ingredients; mixing well.

2. Stir in pecans and mix until pecans are well coated.

3. Pour equal amounts into each pie crust. Bake at 350F for 40 to 45 min. or until center of pie is slightly firm.

Recommend 1 medium slice per serving

===

CHERRY PIE

1 Can	-	Cherry pie filling (No Sugar)
1/2 Cup	-	Splenda Sugar Blend for Baking
1 Tbsp.	-	Cornstarch
1 Tbsp.	-	Light Margarine (soften)
1 Tbsp.	-	Vanilla
1	-	Egg
2 (9 inch)	-	Uncooked Pie Crust

Preparation: Preheat oven 375F

1. In small bowl mix cornstarch and splenda sugar, mix until well blended.

2. Pour cherry filling into medium bowl add cornstarch mixture and vanilla. Mix until well blended (do not beat).

3. Pour mixture into pie crust, place pinches or margarine all over pie filling.

4. Place second pie crust over filling, pinch edges together to seal. Cut 4 slits in top of crust. Beat egg and brush over top of crust. Bake at 375F 40 to 45 min. or until golden brown.

Recommend 1 medium slice per serving

LEMON CUSTARD PIE

1/2 Stick	-	Light Butter
1 Tbsp.	-	All Purpose Flour
3/4 Cup	-	Splenda Sugar Blend for Baking
1/3 Cup	-	Lemon Juice
1/3 Cup	-	Half & Half Milk
5	-	Eggs

Preparation: Preheat oven 350F

1. Melt butter in microwave; set aside. Combine flour and splenda mix well. Whisk eggs and sugar mixture in medium bowl until blended. Slowly add half & half and lemon juice mix until well blended.

2. Pour into pie crust and bake for 45 min or until lightly brown.

Recommend 1 medium slice per serving

===

BLUEBERRY PIE

9 inch	-	2 Pie Crust (buy Crust)
1 Can	-	Blueberry Pie Filling (NO SUGAR)
1/2 Cup	-	Splenda Sugar Blend for Baking
1 Tbsp.	-	Cornstarch
1 Tbsp.	-	Light Margarine (soften)
1 Tbsp.	-	Vanilla
1	-	Egg

Preparation: Preheat oven 375F

1. In small bowl, mix cornstarch and splenda sugar, mix until well blended.

2. Pour blueberry filling into medium bowl; add cornstarch mixture to filling, add vanilla. Mix until well blended. (DO NOT BEAT)

3. Pour blueberry mixture into pie crust; place pinches of margarine all over filling.

4. Place second pie crust over filling; pinch edges together to seal. Cut 4 openings in top of crust.

5. Beat egg and brush over top of crust. Bake at 375F 40 to 50 min. or until golden brown.

Recommend 1 medium slice per serving

APPLE PIE

9 inch	-	2 Pie Crust (buy Crust)
1 Can	-	Apple Pie Filling (NO SUGAR)
1/2 Cup	-	Splenda Sugar Blend for Baking
1 Tbsp.	-	Cornstarch
1 Tsp.	-	Cinnamon
1 Tbsp.	-	Light Margarine (soften)
1 Tbsp.	-	Vanilla
1	-	Egg

Preparation: Preheat oven 375F

1. In small bowl, mix cornstarch, cinnamon and splenda, mix until well blended.

2. Pour apple filling into medium bowl; cut apples into small pieces, add cornstarch mixture and vanilla. Mix until well blended. (DO NOT BEAT)

3. Pour apple mixture into pie crust; place pinches of margarine all over filling.

4. Place second pie crust over filling; pinch edges together to seal. Cut 4 opening in top of crust.

5. Beat egg and brush over top of crust. Bake at 375F 40 to 50 min. or until golden brown.

Recommend 1 medium slice per serving

PEACH PIE

9 inch	-	2 Pie Crust (buy Crust)
1 Can	-	Peach Pie Filling (NO SUGAR)
1/2 Cup	-	Splenda Sugar Blend for Baking
1 Tbsp.	-	Cornstarch
1 Tsp.	-	Cinnamon
1 Tbsp.	-	Light Margarine (soften)
1 Tbsp.	-	Vanilla
1	-	Egg

Preparation: Preheat oven 375F

1. In small bowl, mix cornstarch, cinnamon, and splenda, mix until well blended.

2. Pour peach filling into medium bowl; add cornstarch mixture and vanilla. Mix until well blended. (DO NOT BEAT)

3. Pour peach mixture into pie crust; place pinches of margarine over filling.

4. Place second pie crust over filling; pinch edges together to seal. Cut 4 opening in top of crust.

5. Beat egg and brush over top of crust. Bake at 375F 40 to 50 min. or until golden brown.

Recommend 1 medium slice per serving

BLUEBERRY CHEESECAKE PIE

1 (8 oz.) Pkg.	-	Cream Cheese (Fat Free)
1 Cup	-	Splenda Sugar Blend for Baking (Divided)
1/2 Cup	-	Sour Cream (Low Fat)
1 Tbsp.	-	Lemon Juice
1 1/2 Tbsp.	-	Cornstarch
1	-	Graham Cracker Crust (Reduce Fat)
1 Can	-	Blueberry pie filling (NO SUGAR)
1	-	Egg

Preparation: Preheat oven 325F

1. In small bowl, combine splenda sugar and cornstarch. Mix until well blended. Save 1/2 Cup of mixture for topping.

2. Mix cream cheese in mixing bowl; add 1/2 Cup splenda and cornstarch mixture, beat well. Add sour cream and lemon juice.

3. Add egg and mix until well blended. Pour into graham crust and bake at 325F for approx. 30 to 40 min.

BLUEBERRY TOPPING

1. Pour blueberry pie filling in saucepan adding remaining splenda and cornstarch mixture. Mix and heat until mixture comes to a boil. Remove from heat and let cool. When cream cheese pie has cooled spoon mixture on top of pie.

2. Place in refrigerator for approx. 4 hours before serving.

Recommend 1 medium slice per serving

CHERRY CHEESECAKE PIE

1 (8 oz.) Pkg.	-	Cream Cheese (Low Fat)
1/2 Cup	-	Sour Cream (Low Fat)
1	-	Egg
1/2 Cup	-	Splenda Sugar Blend for Baking
1 1/2 Tbsp.	-	Cornstarch
1 Tbsp.	-	Lemon Juice
1	-	Egg
1	-	Graham Cracker Crust (Reduced Fat)
FILLING		
1 Can	-	Cherry pie filling (NO SUGAR)
1/2 Cup	-	Splenda Sugar Blend for Baking
1 Tbsp.	-	Cornstarch

Preparation: Preheat oven at 350F

1. Beat cream cheese in bowl; in small bowl blend cornstarch and splenda. Add to cream cheese; blend until smooth.

2. Add sour cream, lemon juice and egg; mix until blended. Pour into graham cracker crust and bake approx. 40 min.

FILLING

1. Blend cornstarch and splenda in small bowl. In saucepan add pie filling; fold in splenda mixture; do not beat. Simmer over low heat until splenda has dissolved.

2. When pie and filling has completely cooled add filling to cream cheese and refrigerate approx. 3 hrs. before serving.

Recommend 1 medium slice per serving

STRAWBERRY CHEESECAKE PIE

1 (8 oz.) Pkg.	-	Cream Cheese (Fat Free)
1 Cup	-	Splenda Sugar Blend for Baking (Divided)
1/2 Cup	-	Sour Cream (Low Fat)
1 Tbsp.	-	Lemon Juice
1 1/2 Tsp.	-	Cornstarch
1	-	Graham Cracker Crust (Reduce Fat)
1 Can	-	Strawberry pie filling (NO SUGAR)
1	-	Egg

Preparation: Preheat oven 325F

1. In small bowl, combine splenda sugar and cornstarch. Mix until well blended. Save 1/2 Cup mixture for topping.

2. Mix cream cheese in mixing bowl; add 1/2 Cup splenda and cornstarch mixture, beat well. Add sour cream and lemon juice.

3. Add egg and mix until well blended. Pour into graham crust and bake at 325F for approx. 30 to 40 min.

STRAWBERRY TOPPING

1. Pour strawberry pie filling in saucepan adding remaining splenda and cornstarch mixture. Mix and heat until mixture comes to a boil. Remove from heat and let cool. When cream cheese pie has cooled spoon mixture on top of pie.

2. Place in refrigerator for approx. 4 hours before serving.

Recommend 1 medium slice per serving

SWEET POTATO PIE

4 Cups	-	Sweet Potatoes (cooked)
2/3 Cup	-	Water
1 1/2 Cups	-	Splenda Sugar Blend for Baking
2/3 Cup	-	Half & Half Milk
1 Tsp.	-	Cinnamon
1/2 Tsp.	-	Nutmeg
2 Tbsp.	-	Lemon Juice
1 Tbsp.	-	Vanilla
4	-	Eggs
1 Stick	-	Land O Lakes Light Butter
2 (9")	-	Pie Crust (Buy your crust)

Preparation: Preheat oven 350F

1. Poke holes in pie crust with fork along bottom and sides. Place in oven and bake approx. 10 min. Remove and set aside.

2. Peel and cut up potatoes in 1/4 inch pieces. Simmer in 2/3 Cup water until very tender. Drain and place in large mixing bowl. Add cut up butter and mix well. Add remaining ingredients blend with mixer on medium speed until very smooth.

4. Pour mixture in 2 pie crust and bake at 350F for approx. 40 min. or until pie is firm in center.

Recommend 1 medium slice per serving

CHERRY COBBLER

1 Can	-	Cherries (No Sugar) Pie Filling
2 Tbsp.	-	Light Margarine
1 Tsp.	-	Baking Powder
1 Tsp.	-	Vanilla
1/2 Cup	-	Swans Down Cake Flour
2/3 Cup	-	Splenda Sugar Blend for Baking
1/2 Cup	-	Half & Half Milk
1	-	Egg

Preparation: Preheat oven 350F

1. Melt margarine in deep pie dish. Spoon cherries along the bottom of pie dish. Sprinkle 1/4 Cup splenda sugar over top of cherries.

2. In large measuring Cup combine flour, baking powder and 1/2 Cup splenda sugar blend well.

3. Add half & half, vanilla and egg to flour mixture, beat until smooth. Pour mixture over cherries making sure all cherries are covered with batter. Bake at 350F for 40 min. Turn oven to broil to brown.

Recommend 1/2 Cup per serving

BLUEBERRY COBBLER

1 Can	-	Blueberry (No Sugar) Pie Filling
2 Tbsp.	-	Light Margarine
1 Tsp.	-	Baking Powder
1 Tsp.	-	Vanilla
1/2 Cup	-	Swans Down Cake Flour
2/3 Cup	-	Splenda Sugar Blend for Baking
1/2 Cup	-	Half & Half Milk
1	-	Egg

Preparation: Preheat oven 350F

1. Melt margarine in deep pie dish. Spoon berries along the bottom of pie dish. Sprinkle 1/4 Cup splenda sugar over top of berries.

2. In large measuring Cup combine flour, baking powder and 1/2 Cup splenda sugar blend well.

3. Add half & half, vanilla and egg to flour mixture, beat until smooth. Pour mixture over berries making sure all berries are covered with batter. Bake at 350F for 40 min. Turn oven to broil to brown.

Recommend 1/2 Cup per serving

LEMON DELIGHT

2 1/2 Cups	-	Swans Down Cake Flour
2 Sticks	-	Land O Lakes (Light Butter) soften
1 1/2 Cups	-	Splenda Sugar Blend for Baking
1 Cup	-	Fat Free Milk
1 Tbsp.	-	Baking Powder
1/4 Tsp.	-	Baking Soda
1 Tbsp.	-	Vanilla Extract
3 Tbsp.	-	Lemon Juice
5	-	Egg Yolks

Preparation:

1. Combine cake flour, baking powder, baking soda, and splenda sugar; mix with spoon until well blended.

2. Cut soft butter into chunks add to flour mixture. Mix at medium speed until mixture is crumbly approx. 1 min.

3. Pour 1/4 Cup milk into flour mixture, mix at low speed approx. 30 sec. Add remaining milk, lemon juice, egg yolks and vanilla mix for 30 sec. Scrap sides, turn blender to high and mix approx. 1 1/2 minutes.

4. Spray two (2) 9" cake pans with (cooking spray with flour) and pour cake batter evenly in pan. Shake pan to even out batter.

5. Bake at 350F approx. 30 to 40 min. or until toothpick comes out clean.

ICING

1/2 Cup	-	Lemon Juice
1/2 Cup	-	Splenda Sugar Blend for Baking
1 Tsp.	-	Cornstarch
1 (8 oz.) Tube	-	Fat Free Whip Cream (Thawed)

Preparation:

1. In small bowl combine splenda sugar and cornstarch mix well. In small saucepan combine splenda mixture and lemon juice. Simmer over low heat until mixture comes to light boil. Remove and pour in large mixing bowl. Let cool.

2. When completely cooled fold in thawed whip cream (do not beat) mix well making sure whip cream is well blended. Spread on cake.

Recommend 1 medium slice per serving

COCO DELIGHT CAKE

2 1/2 Cups	-	Swans Down Cake Flour
2 Sticks	-	Land O Lakes (Light Butter) soften
1 1/2 Cups	-	Splenda Sugar Blend for Baking
1 Cup	-	Fat Free Milk
1 Tbsp.	-	Baking Powder
1/4 Tsp.	-	Baking Soda
1 Tbsp.	-	Vanilla Extract
1/3 Cup	-	Coco
5	-	Egg Yolks

Preparation:

1. Combine cake flour, baking powder, baking soda, splenda sugar, and coco; mix with spoon until well blended.

2. Cut soft butter into chunks add to flour mixture. Mix at medium speed until mixture is crumble approx. 1 min.

3. Pour 1/4 Cup milk into flour mixture, mix at low speed approx. 30 sec. Add remaining milk, egg yolks and vanilla mix for 30 sec. Scrap sides, turn blender to high and mix approx 1 1/2 minutes.

4. Spray two (2) 9" cake pans with (cooking spray with flour) and pour cake batter evenly in pan. Shake pan to even out batter.

5. Bake at 350F approx. 30 to 40 min. or until toothpick comes out clean.

COCO DELIGHT ICING

1/2 Cup	-	Coco
1/2 Stick	-	Land O Lakes (light butter)
2/3 Cup	-	Splenda Sugar Blend for Baking
1/2 Cup	-	Half & Half Milk
1 Tsp.	-	Cornstarch
1 Tbsp.	-	Vanilla
1 (8 oz.) Tube	-	Fat Free Whip Cream (Thawed)

Preparation:

1. In medium saucepan combine butter and half & half, heat until butter is melted. Combine coco, splenda sugar and cornstarch, mix well.

2. Add coco mixture to butter mixture heat until mixture comes to a light boil, stirring occasionally. Remove from heat add vanilla and pour in large bowl and let cool.

3. When completely cooled, blend on medium with mixture until creamery. Fold in thawed whip cream (do not beat). Blend well making sure whip cream is well blended. Spread over cold cake.

Recommend 1 medium slice per serving

STRAWBERRY SHORTCAKE

2 1/2 Cups	-	Swans Down Cake Flour
2 Sticks	-	Land O Lakes (Light Butter) soften
1 1/2 Cups	-	Splenda Sugar Blend for Baking
1 Cup	-	Fat Free Milk
1 Tbsp.	-	Baking Powder
1/4 Tsp.	-	Baking Soda
1 Tbsp.	-	Vanilla Extract
5	-	Egg Yolks

Preparation:

1. Combine cake flour, baking powder, baking soda, and splenda sugar; mix with spoon until well blended.

2. Cut soft butter into chunks add to flour mixture. Mix at medium speed until mixture is crumbly approx. 1 min.

3. Pour 1/4 Cup milk into flour mixture, mix at low speed approx. 30 sec. Add remaining milk, egg yolks and vanilla mix for 30 sec. Scrap sides, turn blender to high and mix approx. 1 1/2 minutes.

4. Spray 13 x 9 x 2 pan with (cooking spray with flour) and pour cake batter evenly in pan. Drop pan on counter to even out batter.

5. Bake at 350F approx. 30 to 40 min. or until toothpick comes out clean.

ICING

1 Cup	-	Smuckers Strawberry Preserves (No Sugar)
1/2 Cup	-	Splenda Sugar Blend for Baking
1 (8 oz.) Tub	-	Fat Free Whip Cream (Thawed)

Preparation:

1. In small saucepan combine splenda and strawberry preserves. Simmer over low heat until mixture comes to light boil. Stir occasionally. Pour in large bowl and let cool. Fold whip cream in strawberry mixture and mix well.

2. When completely cooled, pour strawberry mixture over entire cake. Spread evenly making sure cake is covered with strawberries.

3. Cut into squares and serve with whip cream.

Recommend 1 medium slice per serving

APRICOT CAKE

2 1/2 Cups	-	Swans Down Cake Flour
2 Sticks	-	Land O Lakes (Light Butter) soften
1 1/2 Cups	-	Splenda Sugar Blend for Baking
1 Cup	-	Fat Free Milk
1 Tbsp.	-	Baking Powder
1/4 Tsp.	-	Baking Soda
1 Tbsp.	-	Vanilla Extract
5	-	Egg Yolks

Preparation:

1. Combine cake flour, baking powder, baking soda, and splenda sugar; mix with spoon until well blended.

2. Cut soft butter into chunks add to flour mixture. Mix at medium speed until mixture is crumbly approx. 1 min.

3. Pour 1/4 Cup milk into flour mixture, mix at low speed approx. 30 sec. Add remaining milk, egg yolks and vanilla mix for 30 sec. Scrap sides, turn blender to high and mix approx. 1 1/2 minutes.

4. Spray two (2) 9" cake pans with (cooking spray with flour) and pour cake batter evenly in pan. Shake pan to even out cake.

5. Bake at 350F approx. 30 to 40 min. or until toothpick comes out clean.

ICING

1 Cup	-	Smuckers Apricot Preserves (No Sugar)
1/2 Cup	-	Splenda Sugar Blend for Baking
1 (8 oz.) Tub	-	Fat Free Whip Cream (Thawed)

Preparation:

1. In small saucepan combine splenda and apricot preserves. Simmer over low heat until mixture comes to a light boil. Stir occasionally. Pour in large bowl and let cool.

2. When completely cooled, fold in soft whip cream (Do Not Beat), mix well making sure whip cream is well blended. Spread on cake.

Recommend 1 medium slice per serving

ORANGE CAKE

2 1/2 Cups	-	Swans Down Cake Flour
2 Sticks	-	Land O Lakes (Light Butter) soften
1 1/2 Cups	-	Splenda Sugar Blend for Baking
1 Cup	-	Fat Free Milk
1/3 Cup	-	Orange Juice
1 Tbsp.	-	Baking Powder
1/4 Tsp.	-	Baking Soda
1 Tbsp.	-	Vanilla Extract
5	-	Egg yolks

Preparation:

1. Combing cake flour, baking powder, baking soda, and splenda sugar; mix with spoon until well blended.

2. Cut soft butter into chunks add to flour mixture. Mix at medium speed until mixture is crumbly approx. 1 min.

3. Pour 1/4 Cup milk into flour mixture, mix at low speed approx. 30 sec. Add remaining milk, orange juice, egg yolks and vanilla mix for 30 sec. Scrap sides, turn blender to high and mix approx. 1 1/2 minutes.

4. Spray two (2) 9" cake pans with (cooking spray with flour) and pour cake batter evenly in pan. Shake pan to even out cake.

5. Bake at 350F approx. 30 to 40 min. or until toothpick comes out clean.

ICING

1 Cup	-	Smuckers Orange Preserves (No Sugar)
1/2 Cup	-	Splenda Sugar Blend for Baking
1 (8 oz.) Tub	-	Fat Free Whip Cream (Thawed)

Preparation:

1. In small saucepan combine splenda and orange preserves. Simmer over low heat until mixture comes to light boil. Stir occasionally. Pour in large bowl and let cool.

2. When completely cooled, fold in soft whip cream (Do Not Beat), mix well making sure whip cream is well blended. Spread on cake.

Recommend 1 medium slice per serving

BANANA PUDDING

1 Box	-	Vanilla Sugar Free Jell-O Pudding
2 Cups	-	Half & Half Milk
1 Tsp.	-	Vanilla
1/3 Cup	-	Splenda Sugar Blend for Baking
1 Tbsp.	-	Lemon Juice
4	-	Bananas
25	-	Vanilla Wafers (Reduced Fat)

Preparation:

1. In medium saucepan; combine half & half and pudding with wire whisk over low heat.

2. Add splenda sugar stirring constantly until mixture comes to a boil. Add lemon juice and remove from heat.

3. In medium casserole dish add a layer of cookies and cut up 2 bananas over cookies, pour half of milk mixture over bananas and cookies. Repeat cookies, bananas and pudding.

4. Serve warm or cold.

Recommend 1/2 Cup per serving

===

CHOCOLATE WALNUTS

1/2 Cup	-	Heavy Cream
1 Tbsp.	-	Light Margarine
1 Tbsp.	-	Splenda Sugar Blend for Baking
1 (12oz.) Pkg.	-	Semi Sweet Chocolate Morsels
2 Cups	-	Walnuts or Pecans
1 Tbsp.	-	Vanilla

Preparation:

1. In medium saucepan add cream, margarine, splenda and chocolate morsels. Simmer over low heat until morsels have completely melted.

2. Remove from heat add nuts and vanilla, mix until all nuts are completely covered with chocolate. Pour into baking pan or casserole dish. Refrigerate approx. 2 hrs. Cut into 2 inch squares and serve.

Recommend 1 square per serving

TRAIL MIX

1 Cup	-	Walnuts
1 Cup	-	Pecans (whole)
1 Cup	-	Sunflower Seeds
1 Tbsp.	-	House Seasoning
1 Tbsp.	-	Low Fat Oil
1 Tsp.	-	Splenda Sugar Blend for Baking

Preparation: Preheat oven 400F

1. In a large bowl add nuts and sunflower seeds. Sprinkle with low fat oil, house seasoning and splenda sugar. Toss until nuts are well coated.

2. Spread nuts on large baking sheet making sure nuts are not stacked. Bake approx. 10 min. Remove and serve.

3. Store in large jar for snacking.

Recommend 1/2 Cup per serving

Miscellaneous

CHEESE CORNBREAD

1 Cup	-	Plain Yellow Cornmeal
1/2 Cup	-	All Purpose Flour
2 Tbsp.	-	Splenda Sugar Blend for Baking
1 Tbsp.	-	Light Margarine
1 Tbsp.	-	Baking Powder
1	-	Egg
1/2 Cup	-	Cheddar Cheese (Reduced Fat)
2/3 Cup	-	Half & Half Milk

Preparation: Preheat oven 350F

1. Combine all the above ingredients (except margarine) Mix until well blended.

2. Melt margarine in a non-stick pan add batter and bake 30 to 40 min or until golden brown.

Recommend 1 medium slice per serving

CORNBREAD DRESSING

2 Cups	-	Plain Yellow Cornmeal
1 Cup	-	All Purpose Flour
1/2 Cup	-	Half & Half Milk
1 Cup	-	Chicken Broth
4	-	Eggs (Slightly Beaten)
2 Tbsp.	-	Baking Powder
1 Tbsp.	-	Low Fat Oil

Preparation: Preheat oven 350F

1. In large bowl combine all the above ingredients. Mix well. Pour into greased pan and bake 35 to 40 min. or until golden brown.

==

SEASONING

5 Sticks	-	Celery (chopped)
1 lg.	-	Onion (chopped)
1 lg.	-	Green Pepper (chopped)
1 Bunch	-	Green Onion (chopped)
2	-	Chicken Bouillon Cubes
4 Tbsp.	-	Light Margarine
4	-	Eggs
1 1/2 Tbsp.	-	Poultry Seasoning
1 Can	-	Cream of Mushroom Soup
2 Cans	-	Cream of Chicken Soup
2 Cans	-	Chicken Broth (Low Sodium)

1. In large saucepan add chopped onions, celery, peppers, chicken bouillon cubes, light margarine and 1 Cup water. Simmer until tender.

2. In large bowl crumble cornbread into small pieces, add celery mixture, eggs, poultry seasoning, soups and broth. Mix well to blend all the ingredients together.

3. Pour in large baking dish and bake at 350F until firm approx. 1 hour. (SAVE 2 CUPS FOR GIBBLET GRAVY)

Recommend 1/2 Cup per serving

CHEESE GRITS

1 1/3 Cups	-	Water
1/3 Cup	-	Grits
1/4 Cup	-	Heavy Cream
1/2 Cup	-	Cheddar Cheese (Reduced Fat)
2 Tbsp.	-	Light Margarine

Preparation:

1. Bring water, margarine to a boil, stir in grits, cover and reduce heat. Stir occasionally to eliminate sticking.

2. Simmer approx. 15 min. and add cream and cheese, allow cheese to melt and serve.

Recommend 1/2 Cup per serving

==

GRITS

1 1/3 Cups	-	Water
1/3 Cup	-	Grits
1 Cube	-	Chicken Bouillon
2 Tbsp.	-	Light Margarine

Preparation:

1. Bring water, margarine and bouillon cube to a boil, stir in grits cover and reduce heat. Stir occasionally to eliminate sticking.

2. Simmer approx. 15 min. Mix well and serve.

Recommend 1/2 Cup per serving

PECAN PANCAKES

1 Cup	-	Whole Wheat Flour
1/2 Cup	-	Fat Free Milk
1/2 Cup	-	Pecans or walnuts
1 Tbsp.	-	Splenda Sugar Blend for Baking
1 Tbsp.	-	Baking Powder
1	-	Egg

Preparation:

1. Heat skillet or griddle, add 1 teaspoon low fat oil. Combine all the above ingredients, mix until well blended.

2. Pour batter on hot griddle and brown on each side. Add 1 teaspoon low fat oil for each new batch of pancakes.

3. Serve with sugar free syrup.

Recommend 2 small pancakes per serving

===

CHEESE PANCAKES

1 Cup	-	Whole Wheat Flour
1/2 Cup	-	Fat Free Milk
1/2 Cup	-	Cheddar Cheese (Reduced Fat)
1 Tbsp.	-	Splenda Sugar Blend for Baking
1 Tbsp.	-	Baking Powder
1	-	Egg

Preparation:

1. Heat skillet or griddle, add 1 teaspoon low fat oil. Combine all the above ingredients, mix until well blended.

2. Pour batter on hot griddle and brown on each side. Add 1 teaspoon low fat oil for each new batch of pancakes.

3. Serve with sugar free syrup.

Recommend 2 small pancakes per serving

REFERENCE NOTES

1. **Blood Pressure Chart** - http://cmbi.bjmu.eda.cn/heart-news/ hypgquide042199ht
2. **Cholesterol Chart** - www.onlinebangalore.com/heal/blo-cho.htm
3. **Diabetes Chart** - Lifescan, Inc. 1999 (AW052-289-01E)
4. **Weight Charts** - www.usmilitary.about.com/library/milinfo/arfitness/ blarfitness.htm
5. **Total Fat Charts** - American Diabetes Assoc.
6. **Portion Sizes** - American Diabetes Assoc.
7. **Proper Foot Care** - SB Smith Kline Beecham Pharmaceuticals

IMPORTANT NUMBERS

1. American Diabetes Association   1-800-342-2383
     www.diabetes.org

2. American Stroke Association   1-888-478-7653
     www.strokeassociation.org

3. American Heart Association   1-800-242-8721
     www.americanheart.org

4. American Cancer Society   1-800-227-2345
     www.cancer.org

These are amazing organizations
and are more than happy to assist you in any way they can.

Index

ABOUT THE AUTHOR

E.L. Hughes was born in the South and has always been interested in cooking. Southern born and bred, we are accustomed to delicious foods that burst with flavor.

When my husband was diagnosed with diabetes, high blood pressure and heart failure, cooking for the family became a difficult task.

Meal time was depressing, my husband meals were bland and unsatisfying, most of the time he wouldn't eat. This is when I decided to find ways to "spice-up" his meals.

It's a timely question: How can you prepare healthy meals for a person who have spent a lifetime eating good old Southern cooking? So the dilemma began. By trail and error, I developed recipes without salt or sugar that the whole family could enjoy eating.

This book truly serves many purposes. It allows the restricted family member to enjoy the same meals the rest of the family enjoys at meal time. It will also save the meal preparer time. No longer will two meals have to be prepared.

The cooking methods in this book are designed to create healthy meals without sacrificing flavor.